THE F.R.E.E.D.O.M. PROTOCOL
PROTOCOL

Dr. Paul Fisher, D.C.
The F.R.E.E.D.O.M. Protocol

Published by Spines
ISBN: 979-8-89691-163-0

THE F.R.E.E.D.O.M. PROTOCOL

TRANSFORMING KNEE PAIN INTO STRENGTH

DR. PAUL FISHER, D.C.

CONTENTS

FOREWORD

As a fellow chiropractor and someone who's spent years
studying the intricacies of the human body, I've seen
firsthand the debilitating effects of knee pain. It robs
people of their mobility, their joy, and their freedom to
live life fully. I've also witnessed the transformative
power of the right approach – a power that Dr. Paul
Fisher, D.C., captures brilliantly in "The F.R.E.E.D.O.M.
Protocol."

Paul and I are colleagues, both members of the Driven
Doc community at The Data Driven Practice. But
beyond that, we're united by a shared passion:
empowering people to take control of their health.
Paul's F.R.E.E.D.O.M. Protocol is more than just a
program; it's a philosophy. It's a testament to the fact
that knee pain doesn't have to be a life sentence. It's a

blueprint for reclaiming strength, mobility, and the sheer joy of movement.

This book is a gift to anyone who's ever struggled with knee pain. It's a beacon of hope, offering a proven, non-invasive path to healing. It's also a testament to the expertise of Dr. Fisher and his dedicated team at Innovative Nerve & Joint Centers. If you're ready to break free from the chains of knee pain, this book is your guide. It's time to discover the freedom that awaits you.

Dr. Cory Frogley, D.C.
Co-Founder, The Data Driven Practice

DISCLAIMER

The information provided in this book is intended for educational purposes only and is not a substitute for professional medical advice. The author and publisher are not liable for any adverse effects or consequences resulting from the use of the information presented herein. All testimonials found in this book are not typical, and individual results may vary. Always consult your physician or a qualified healthcare provider regarding any health concerns or before making any decisions related to your health or treatment.

Results may vary based on individual conditions and adherence to the recommended care plan. No guarantees of a cure or specific results are implied. Testimonials reflect individual patient experiences and are not indicative of guaranteed outcomes for all patients. The consultation is intended to assess your condition and determine potential options, but no specific treatment outcome is guaranteed. This manuscript complies with state advertising regulations and does not imply superiority over other healthcare professionals or methods. Free services, if mentioned, are offered without any condition of additional purchase. Please consult with Dr. Paul Fisher, D.C., for a personalized assessment of your health.

ABOUT THE AUTHOR

I'm Dr. Paul Fisher, D.C., and I understand the frustration of chronic knee pain. I suffered with it myself. After blowing out my ACL, MCL and meniscus on my right knee in high school, its never been the same. For years, (decades really), it would bother me on stairs, long runs, snowboarding or kneeling. Perhaps most frustratingly when I was sitting, not doing anything at all! I'd done my PT, laser, stim, creams, you name it. And everything worked. Sorta... I've seen the way it can erode your physical freedom and diminish your quality of life. While traditional medicine often relies on painkillers and temporary solutions, I believe a better path exists – a path to true healing. And I was determined to find it.

My own journey into healthcare wasn't straightforward. Originally, I majored in Management Information Systems. Yet, an underlying thirst for knowledge about the human body led me to pivot. With extensive chiropractic training, a Master's in Nutrition, and advanced certifications, I've gained a deep understanding of how the body functions, heals, and sometimes falters. My experiences at the National Naval Medical Hospital further reinforced the importance of an integrated approach to treatment.

My studies and clinical work have solidified my belief that knee pain, and many other chronic issues, often stem from hidden causes that need to be addressed to achieve lasting results. That's why I developed the F.R.E.E.D.O.M. Protocol. This comprehensive approach is designed to not only relieve your pain but also empower you to reclaim the strength and mobility you may think are gone forever.

At the Innovative Nerve & Joint Centers, finding the root cause of your health challenges is our priority. I want you to feel your absolute best, and we will work tirelessly to help you get there. When I'm not with patients, I'm most likely pursuing more knowledge, grilling up something delicious, or coaching my son's teams.

Let's begin your journey towards a pain-free life!

1

———

UNDERSTANDING KNEE PAIN

The waiting room was quiet, except for the gentle hum of the air purifier and the rhythmic tap-tap-tapping of my pen against my notepad. I was reviewing Maggie's file, a smile tugging at the corners of my mouth. Just a few months ago, she'd walked into my office, her face etched with pain and a palpable sense of hopelessness. Knee pain had stolen her joy, transforming her daily walks with her beloved golden retriever, Gus, into a torturous ordeal. She'd tried everything – physical therapy, injections, even considered surgery – but nothing seemed to provide lasting relief. "I'm starting to think I'll never be able to enjoy a simple walk again," she'd confessed, her voice thick with emotion.

We started Maggie on the FREEDOM Protocol, and the transformation has been nothing short of remarkable.

Her initial assessment revealed significant muscle imbalances and limitations in her range of motion. We created a tailored plan, focusing on strengthening her core, improving her hip mobility, and correcting her gait. We also incorporated cutting-edge therapies like cold laser and Trigenics® to address inflammation and neuromuscular dysfunction.

Today, Maggie practically skipped into my office, Gus trotting happily beside her. "Dr. Fisher," she beamed, "I can't believe the difference! I'm walking pain-free, further than I have in years. Gus and I are finally back to our old routines, enjoying those long walks in the park. My experience with the FREEDOM Protocol has truly changed my life, though I understand that every patient's journey is unique and my success doesn't guarantee similar results for others." Her words, filled with genuine gratitude and a renewed sense of vitality, are a testament to the power of the FREEDOM Protocol.

Maggie's story, while just one example, underscores a critical truth: knee pain doesn't have to be a life sentence. There is hope, and it starts with understanding.

The Silent Epidemic

Knee Pain: A Common Burden

Your knees are remarkable. They're the largest, most complex joints in your body, a marvel of engineering meant to bend, straighten, twist, and bear your weight through a lifetime of movement. It's easy to take them for granted... until they start to hurt.

Knee pain isn't just an annoyance; it's surprisingly common. Millions of people – athletes, office workers, grandparents – struggle with it each year. Yet, we often downplay those early twinges and aches. It's this subtle dismissal that makes knee pain a truly silent epidemic.

The Dangers of Hidden Knee Issues

Take Sarah, a busy mom of three. She noticed her knee felt stiff after running errands, but figured it was just getting older. Months later, the pain was waking her up at night, and simply going up the stairs became a challenge.

Or there's Alex, a college athlete. He shrugged off minor knee soreness as part of the game. Now, that soreness flares up during every practice, and he fears a season-ending injury could be looming.

Sarah and Alex aren't alone. Knee pain creeps in slowly, often masked by our hectic lives. We tell ourselves it'll go away, or it's just a sign of wear and tear.

Perhaps the worst was Kaitlyn, who's knee pain began in high school, continued through her time as a D1 athlete playing volleyball and had gotten to the point where she had to use a cane. At only 29.

The Price of Ignoring Pain

The truth is, ignoring knee pain comes with a price. As discomfort worsens, it starts to chip away at your life. Activities you once loved become difficult or even impossible. Walking the dog, playing with your kids, or even enjoying a night out dancing might feel out of reach. If you have a manual job, it can even stop you from working. The emotional toll – frustration, worry, a sense of lost freedom – can weigh just as heavily as the physical pain.

Worse yet, untreated knee issues often lead to a cascade of problems. You might unknowingly favor one leg over the other, straining your hips and back. Reduced activity can contribute to weight gain, putting even more stress on your joints.

Early Action for Healthy Knees

The good news is, you don't have to accept knee pain as your fate. Here's what you can do right now:

- **Tune in:** Pay attention to your knees. Do they feel stiff first thing in the morning? Ache after standing for too long? Swell during activities? Don't dismiss even minor twinges.
- **Track it:** Keep a simple log. Note when pain occurs, what activities seem to trigger it, and how it feels (sharp, dull, etc.). This helps identify patterns.
- **Don't self-diagnose:** The internet is full of knee pain theories. Seek qualified advice from a doctor or physical therapist who can pinpoint the true cause.

This chapter is just the beginning. Understanding the scope of the problem is the first step toward finding solutions. Let's dive into the root causes of knee pain next, so you can pave the way for lasting relief.

Root Causes of Knee Pain

Think of your knee pain as a whodunnit mystery. The pain itself is the obvious problem, but to truly solve the case, you need to uncover the culprit lurking behind the scenes. In the office we like to say there's pain and then there's problem. They aren't always the same. Let's track down some of the prime suspects:

- **Injuries: The Usual Suspects:** Just like that awkward twist on the tennis court can leave a sore ankle, knee injuries have a nasty habit of lingering. Sprains, strains, torn ligaments – whether they happened during a dramatic fall or from the repeated stress of your daily runs – injuries are a top cause of knee complaints.

- **The Wear and Tear Factor:** Time has a way of roughing things up, and our knees aren't immune. Osteoarthritis, a condition where the joint's cushioning cartilage slowly breaks down, is an incredibly common cause of knee pain, especially as we age. Stiffness, swelling, and a gradual increase in discomfort are its telltale signs.

- **Hidden Contributors: The Plot Twist:** Sometimes, the true source of your knee pain isn't in the knee at all. Think of your body as an interconnected system. A problem like a weak hip can force your knees to compensate, putting them under strain they weren't designed for. Tight muscles, an out-of-whack stride, even fallen arches in your feet can create a ripple effect that ends with those achy knees.

This is why taking a magnifying glass to your whole body, not just your knees, is crucial in your detective work. Once you start connecting the dots, you might uncover a surprising chain of events that led to your current pain, and that's the key to lasting relief.

Success Stories

Knee pain stories aren't always what you expect. Forget the stereotypical athlete sidelined by a ligament tear. The truth is, knee pain can strike anyone, anytime, and often for reasons that defy the textbook. Here are a couple of real-life examples.

Sarah the Runner: A Case of Misalignment

Sarah prided herself on her dedication to running. She'd conquered countless marathons, pushing her body to the limit. But then, a nagging pain settled in her right knee. Worried about a serious injury, she rushed to the doctor. X-rays revealed no major damage, leaving everyone confused. It wasn't until a biomechanical evaluation that the culprit was identified: Sarah's running form. A slight imbalance in her stride was causing her knee to absorb excessive stress with every step. The solution? Targeted physical therapy exercises to correct her form, combined with a running technique overhaul. Within weeks, Sarah was back on the track, pain-free, and with a newfound appreciation for proper biomechanics.

Grandpa Joe: Weakness in Disguise

Joe, a sprightly 72-year-old, loved taking walks with his dog, Sparky. But lately, those walks had become a struggle. His knees ached, making even flat terrain feel like climbing a mountain. He figured it was "just his age" and resigned himself to a less active life. However, during a routine checkup, his doctor noticed something interesting. Joe's core muscles, which provide essential stability, were significantly weakened. This weakness was causing misalignment in his lower body, putting undue strain on his knees. The answer wasn't some fancy procedure or medication. It was a simple, personalized exercise program designed to strengthen his core. Gradually, the walks with Sparky became easier, then enjoyable. Joe's knee pain wasn't a death knell for his activity; it was a message that needed deciphering.

These stories highlight the importance of looking beyond the knee itself. Knee pain can be a symptom, a red flag waving from a deeper issue. Understanding these unexpected connections is key to unlocking a pain-free future.

Early Intervention: The Key to Faster Healing

Imagine this: you're feeling a dull ache in your shoulder. You shrug it off, assuming it's just a minor discomfort. But what if that ache is a warning sign of a bigger problem brewing in your rotator cuff? The same goes for knee pain. While ignoring it might seem like the easier option in the short term, uncovering the root cause early on offers a treasure trove of benefits:

- **Targeted Treatment, Better Results:** Think of it like this: you wouldn't treat a cold with medication for a broken bone, right? The same principle applies to knee pain. If the culprit is a torn meniscus, you'll need a different approach than if it's arthritis. By pinpointing the exact cause, your healthcare provider can tailor a treatment plan specifically designed to address the issue at its core. This targeted approach often leads to faster healing and a higher chance of long-term success.
- **Preventing Future Problems:** Knee pain can sometimes be a domino effect. Left untreated, a seemingly small issue can snowball into more significant problems down the road. For example, if weak core muscles are causing knee pain, ignoring it could eventually lead to instability and potential injury. Early diagnosis

allows you to intervene before these dominoes start to fall, preventing future complications and saving you time, money, and frustration.

- **Empowerment and Ownership of Your Health:** Knowledge is power, especially when it comes to your body. Understanding the root cause of your knee pain puts YOU in control. It allows you to make informed decisions about your treatment plan and actively participate in your healing journey. You'll also be better equipped to prevent future problems by knowing what activities or movements might aggravate your specific condition.

Taking the time to identify the root cause of your knee pain might seem like an extra hurdle at first. But trust me, when it comes to achieving lasting relief and safeguarding your future health, it's a step worth taking.

Decoding Your Knee Pain

Knee pain can feel like a frustrating mystery. The discomfort is there, but the cause remains stubbornly hidden. Thankfully, there are tools at your disposal to crack the knee pain code and unlock the path to healing.

Step 1: The Doctor is In (and Listening)

The journey starts with a visit to a healthcare professional specializing in knees. They'll act as your detective, gathering clues to solve the case. Expect a detailed conversation about your medical history - past injuries, activity levels, and the specifics of your pain. This is your chance to be the star witness, providing as much information as possible.

Step 2: The Physical Exam - Putting You Through Your Paces

Next comes the physical exam. Your doctor will assess your knee's range of motion, check for tenderness, and test its stability. Think of it as a series of tests to pinpoint exactly where the culprit might be hiding.

Step 3: A Deeper Look - Imaging When Needed

In some cases, additional investigation might be required. X-rays can reveal bone issues, while MRIs provide a detailed picture of soft tissues like ligaments and cartilage. These imaging tools are like powerful magnifying glasses, allowing your doctor to see the inner workings of your knee and identify potential problems.

Step 4: Calling in the Specialists - Considering All Angles

Sometimes, a knee specialist like a sports medicine doctor or a physical therapist can offer valuable insights. They might have specific tests or techniques to pinpoint the cause of your pain. Think of them as specialist detectives, brought in to consult on a particularly tricky case.

Remember: This search for answers is a collaborative effort. The more information you share and the more actively you participate in the process, the faster you'll crack the code and unlock the door to a pain-free future. So, don't hesitate to ask questions and voice any concerns you might have. Together, we can solve the mystery of your knee pain and get you back on the path to an active, fulfilling life.

ACTION STEP: Start a daily journal of your symptoms. This will allow you to more accurately sense your level of improvement when starting a neuropathy treatment regimen.

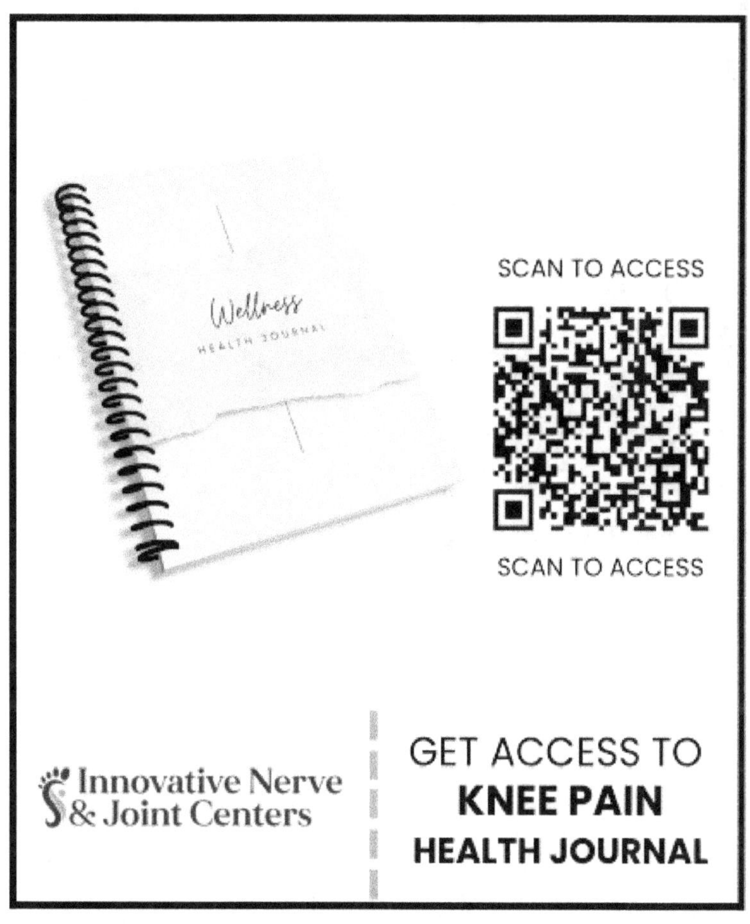

Unlock Your Path To Knee Pain Relief Now: Call (833) 359-6099 To Speak With An Expert Today!

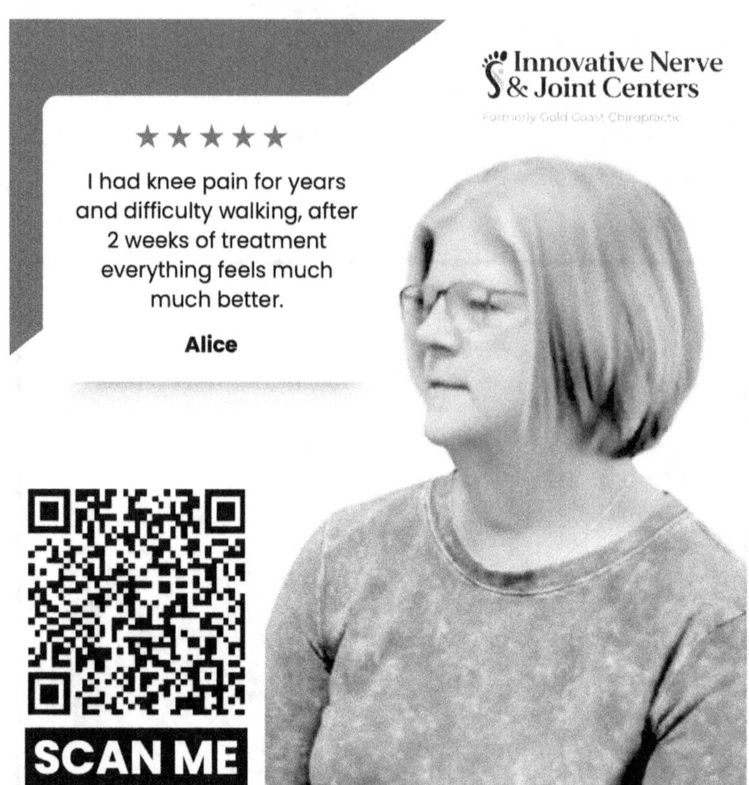
★ ★ ★ ★ ★

I had knee pain for years
and difficulty walking, after
2 weeks of treatment
everything feels much
much better.

Alice

Innovative Nerve
& Joint Centers
Formerly Gold Coast Chiropractic

SCAN ME

THE PROMISE OF THE FREEDOM PROTOCOL

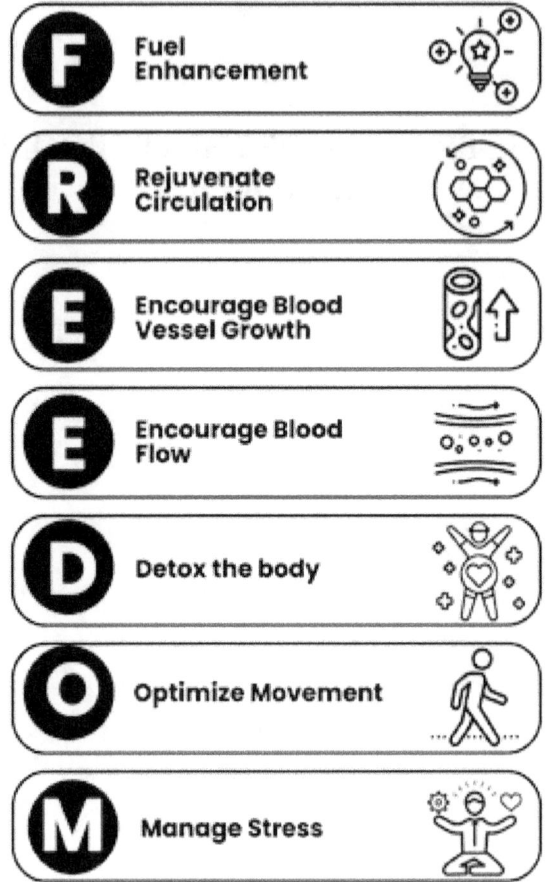

FREEDOM
F — Fuel Enhancement
R — Rejuvenate Circulation
E — Encourage Blood Vessel Growth
E — Encourage Blood Flow
D — Detox the body
O — Optimize Movement
M — Manage Stress

A New Approach to Knee Health

Introducing the FREEDOM Knee Program

If you're ready to kick the frustration of knee pain and reclaim your active life, it's time for something different. The FREEDOM Protocol moves beyond simply treating symptoms. It's a comprehensive plan designed to uncover the true cause of your pain, restore your knees' full potential, and empower you to take charge of your health.

Let's break down the F.R.E.E.D.O.M. acronym:

F: Fuel Enhancement – Your Diet's Power Over Knee Pain

The old saying, "You are what you eat," holds true for your knees, too. The food choices you make every day have a major impact on inflammation in your body, which is often a sneaky culprit behind knee pain.

Think of your body like a high-performance car. If you fill it with low-grade fuel, it won't run smoothly. The same applies to your knees – if you feed them foods high in sugar, processed fats, and inflammatory ingredients, they're going to protest.

But what if you flipped the script? What if you started nourishing your body with foods that naturally reduce inflammation, promote healing, and give your knees the best possible environment to recover?

The Anti-Inflammatory Powerhouse

That's where the "Fuel Enhancement" aspect of the FREEDOM Protocol comes in. It's about making strategic swaps in your diet to:

- **Reduce Inflammation:** Foods rich in omega-3 fatty acids (found in fatty fish like salmon), colorful fruits and veggies (packed with antioxidants), and spices like turmeric and ginger can help calm the flames of inflammation in your joints.
- **Support Joint Health:** Bone broth, leafy greens, and nuts provide nutrients like collagen, vitamin K, and magnesium – essential building blocks for healthy cartilage and strong bones.
- **Optimize Weight:** Excess weight places extra strain on your knees. By focusing on whole, nutrient-dense foods, you'll be better equipped to reach and maintain a healthy weight, which can significantly ease knee pain.

Not Just What You Eat, But How You Eat

Beyond the specific foods, consider *how* you're eating:

- **Stay Hydrated:** Water is crucial for joint lubrication and overall health. Aim to drink plenty throughout the day.
- **Mindful Eating:** Slow down, savor your food, and listen to your body's hunger cues.
- **Meal Timing:** Some people find that smaller, more frequent meals help with energy levels and manage inflammation.

Your Kitchen is Your Pharmacy

Making small changes to your diet can feel like a powerful medicine for your knees. Remember, this is a journey, not a race. Start by incorporating more anti-inflammatory foods, and slowly eliminate those that might be aggravating your pain.

R: Rejuvenate Circulation – Your Knees' Lifeline

Imagine your knees as a bustling city. Just like any city needs a steady flow of traffic to keep things running smoothly, your knees need healthy blood circulation to thrive. When that circulation slows down, it's like a traffic jam – nutrients and oxygen can't reach their destination, waste products build up, and inflammation takes hold.

The Circulatory Superhighway

The "Rejuvenate Circulation" aspect of the FREEDOM Protocol is about getting that traffic moving again. Think of it as clearing the roads and repairing the bridges so your body's natural healing power can reach your knees.

How We Boost Blood Flow:

- **Hands-On Therapies:** Chiropractic adjustments and massage therapy can gently encourage better blood flow by removing restrictions and improving nerve function.
- **Movement is Medicine:** Regular exercise, even low-impact activities like walking or swimming, helps pump blood to your knees, delivering vital nutrients and oxygen.
- **Temperature Therapy:** Alternating hot and cold packs can stimulate blood vessels to open and close, creating a pumping action that helps flush out waste products.
- **Supplements:** Certain natural supplements like ginger and ginkgo biloba can support healthy circulation.

Why Circulation Matters:

- **Reduced Inflammation:** Increased blood flow helps carry away inflammatory substances, naturally reducing swelling and pain.
- **Faster Healing:** With better circulation, the nutrients needed for tissue repair reach your knees more efficiently, accelerating the healing process.
- **Improved Mobility:** Good circulation helps lubricate joints, making it easier to move and reducing stiffness.
- **Overall Well-Being:** Better circulation not only benefits your knees but also supports your overall health.

Your Heart's Connection to Your Knees

Remember, your heart is the engine that drives your circulatory system. Taking care of your cardiovascular health is essential for healthy knees. That means eating a balanced diet, getting regular exercise, and managing stress.

E: Encourage Blood Vessel Growth – Nurturing Your Knee's Network

Picture this: a network of tiny roads weaving through your knee joint, delivering vital nutrients and oxygen while whisking away waste products. These roads are your blood vessels, and they play a critical role in keeping your knees healthy and pain-free.

Over time, due to injury, wear and tear, or other factors, these tiny roads can become damaged or deteriorate. This can lead to reduced blood flow, which in turn can cause pain, inflammation, and slower healing.

Building New Pathways

The "Encourage Blood Vessel Growth" aspect of the FREEDOM Protocol is about stimulating your body to build new, healthy blood vessels and repair existing ones. It's like adding new lanes to the highway and fixing potholes to ensure smooth traffic flow.

How We Encourage Growth:

- **Targeted Nutrition:** Certain foods and supplements, like those rich in nitric oxide (found in beets and leafy greens), can help promote the formation of new blood vessels.
- **Platelet-Rich Plasma (PRP) Therapy:** This innovative treatment utilizes your body's own platelets, which contain growth factors, to stimulate tissue repair and blood vessel growth.

- **Exercise:** Regular exercise, especially weight-bearing activities, can trigger the body to create new blood vessels in response to the increased demand for oxygen and nutrients.
- **Cold Laser Therapy:** This therapy has been shown to stimulate blood vessel growth in damaged tissues.

The Benefits of Enhanced Blood Flow:

- **Reduced Pain:** Better circulation means less inflammation and a healthier environment for your knees.
- **Faster Healing:** With improved blood flow, nutrients and oxygen can reach your joints more efficiently, speeding up the repair process.
- **Stronger Joints:** New blood vessels bring nourishment to cartilage and other tissues, supporting their overall health and resilience.
- **Increased Energy:** When your knees are well-nourished, you'll have more energy for the activities you love.

Your Body's Amazing Ability to Adapt

It's truly remarkable how our bodies can adapt and create new pathways for healing. By encouraging blood vessel growth, we're essentially giving your knees the tools they need to thrive.

E: Encourage Blood Flow – Keep the River Flowing

Think of your blood vessels as a network of rivers, constantly flowing through your body. In your knees, this flow delivers essential nutrients, oxygen, and healing factors while carrying away waste products and inflammatory substances. When this flow is strong and steady, your knees thrive. But if it becomes sluggish or restricted, it's like a dam forming in the river – leading to stagnation and potential problems.

The Importance of Unimpeded Flow

Encouraging blood flow is essential for maintaining healthy knees. It's about keeping the river of life flowing freely to your joints, nourishing them from the inside out.

How We Encourage Blood Flow:

- **Active Movement:** Regular exercise, even simple activities like walking or gentle stretching, acts as a pump, stimulating blood flow to your knees and flushing out waste products.
- **Massage Therapy:** This hands-on technique

can help release muscle tension and improve circulation in the surrounding tissues.

- **Compression Therapy:** Compression socks or sleeves can gently squeeze your legs, aiding in the upward movement of blood and reducing swelling.
- **Hydrotherapy:** Warm water immersion, such as in a hot tub or bath, can help relax muscles and dilate blood vessels, increasing blood flow to your knees.
- **Elevation:** Raising your legs above your heart for short periods can help reduce swelling and promote better circulation.

The Benefits of Enhanced Blood Flow:

- **Pain Reduction:** Increased blood flow delivers more oxygen and nutrients to your knees, reducing inflammation and easing pain.
- **Improved Mobility:** Better circulation helps lubricate joints, making them move more smoothly and reducing stiffness.
- **Faster Healing:** With optimal blood flow, your body can repair damaged tissues more quickly and efficiently.
- **Overall Joint Health:** When your knees receive a steady supply of nutrients and oxygen,

they're better equipped to stay healthy and resilient.

Your Daily Habits Matter

Beyond specific treatments, your daily habits can significantly impact your circulation. Avoiding prolonged sitting, staying hydrated, and managing stress all contribute to a healthier blood flow.

D: Detox the Body – Clearing the Path for Healing

Imagine your body as a filter. Day in and day out, it encounters various substances – some helpful, others potentially harmful. When your body's natural detoxification systems are overwhelmed, these harmful substances can accumulate, triggering inflammation and hindering healing. This is especially problematic for your knees, as inflammation is often a major contributor to pain and stiffness.

Your Body's Cleanup Crew

The "Detox the Body" aspect of the FREEDOM Protocol is about giving your body's internal cleanup crew a little extra support. It's about creating an environment where your natural detoxification processes can function optimally, allowing your knees to heal more efficiently.

How We Support Detoxification:

- **Hydration:** Water is essential for flushing out toxins. Aim for eight glasses or more per day, especially if you're active.
- **Nutrient-Dense Foods:** Load up on fruits, vegetables, and whole grains. These provide antioxidants and fiber, which aid in detoxification.
- **Limit Processed Foods and Sugar:** These can tax your body's detox systems. Opt for whole, unprocessed foods whenever possible.
- **Herbal Teas:** Certain teas, like dandelion root and milk thistle, have been traditionally used to support liver function.
- **Gentle Movement:** Exercise helps your lymphatic system, a key player in detoxification, drain fluids and remove waste products.

Why Detoxification Matters:

- **Reduced Inflammation:** When your body is efficiently eliminating toxins, it can better manage inflammation, which can ease knee pain.

- **Improved Immune Function:** A healthy detox system supports a strong immune response, helping your body fight off infections and heal more effectively.
- **Increased Energy:** When your body isn't burdened by toxins, you'll have more energy to be active and enjoy life.
- **Overall Well-Being:** Detoxification isn't just about your knees; it supports your overall health and vitality.

A Gentle Approach

It's important to note that we're not talking about extreme detoxes or cleanses here. The FREEDOM Protocol focuses on gentle, sustainable practices that support your body's natural ability to detoxify.

O: Optimize Movement – Reclaim Your Natural Rhythm

Think of your knees as part of a complex symphony of movement. When each part of the orchestra – your muscles, joints, and nerves – works in harmony, the result is smooth, pain-free motion. But when one instrument is out of tune, it can disrupt the entire performance, leading to stiffness, discomfort, and even injury.

Rediscovering Your Body's Movement Symphony

The "Optimize Movement" aspect of the FREEDOM Protocol is about fine-tuning your body's orchestra. It's about identifying those movements that might be contributing to your knee pain and finding ways to retrain your body to move with greater ease and efficiency.

How We Optimize Movement:

- **Targeted Exercises:** We'll work with you to develop a personalized exercise plan that strengthens weak muscles, improves flexibility, and enhances coordination.
- **Gait Analysis:** By analyzing the way you walk, we can identify any imbalances or faulty movement patterns that might be stressing your knees.
- **Corrective Exercises:** These exercises are designed to address specific weaknesses and help you develop healthier movement habits.
- **Proprioception Training:** This involves exercises that improve your body's awareness of its position in space, leading to better balance and coordination.
- **Activity Modification:** We'll help you identify activities that might be aggravating your knee

pain and suggest modifications to make them less stressful.

The Benefits of Optimal Movement:

- **Pain Reduction:** By improving your movement patterns, you can reduce the strain on your knees and alleviate pain.
- **Increased Strength:** Targeted exercises will help strengthen the muscles that support your knees, providing greater stability and resilience.
- **Enhanced Flexibility:** Improved flexibility allows for a greater range of motion and reduces the risk of injury.
- **Improved Function:** With optimal movement, you'll be able to perform daily activities and enjoy your favorite hobbies with greater ease.
- **Confidence:** As you gain control over your movement, you'll feel more confident in your body and its abilities.

Your Body's Innate Wisdom

Your body is incredibly adaptable. By optimizing your movement, we're tapping into its innate wisdom and ability to heal. With the right guidance and support, you can relearn how to move with grace and fluidity, freeing your knees from pain and unlocking a world of possibility.

M: Manage Stress – The Mind-Body Connection for Knee Health

It might surprise you, but stress isn't just a mental burden – it can manifest physically, particularly in your joints. When stress hormones like cortisol flood your body, they trigger inflammation, which can worsen knee pain and slow down healing. Plus, when we're stressed, we often tense up, leading to muscle tightness and imbalances that put extra strain on our knees.

Finding Your Calm

The "Manage Stress" aspect of the FREEDOM Protocol is about recognizing the powerful connection between your mind and body. It's about finding healthy ways to manage stress, so your knees (and your whole body) can thrive.

Stress-Busting Techniques:

- **Mindfulness Meditation:** Taking a few minutes each day to focus on your breath and be present in the moment can reduce stress hormones and promote relaxation.

- **Deep Breathing Exercises:** Deep, slow breaths activate your body's relaxation response, lowering heart rate and easing muscle tension.
- **Yoga and Tai Chi:** These gentle practices combine movement with mindful breathing, helping to reduce stress and improve flexibility.
- **Nature Therapy:** Spending time in nature has a calming effect on both the mind and body.
- **Creative Outlets:** Whether it's painting, writing, or playing music, engaging in creative activities can be a great way to de-stress.
- **Professional Support:** If stress feels overwhelming, consider talking to a therapist or counselor.

The Benefits of Stress Management for Knee Health:

- **Reduced Inflammation:** Lower stress levels translate to less inflammation throughout your body, including your knees.
- **Improved Muscle Function:** Relaxed muscles are less likely to become tight and create imbalances that contribute to knee pain.
- **Better Sleep:** Stress can disrupt sleep, which is essential for healing and recovery. Managing stress can lead to more restful sleep and better overall health.

- **Enhanced Mood:** When you're feeling less stressed, you're more likely to be positive and motivated, which can aid in your knee pain journey.

Stress management isn't just about feeling good mentally; it's a crucial component of your physical healing journey. By taking the time to nurture your mind, you're creating a more supportive environment for your knees to heal and thrive.

With the "M" in FREEDOM, we've now covered all the key elements of this comprehensive approach to knee pain. Remember, each aspect works together to create a synergistic effect, empowering you to overcome pain and reclaim your freedom of movement.

Success Stories: Reclaiming Pain-Free Lives

The true power of the FREEDOM Knee Program lies in its ability to transform lives. Don't just take our word for it – hear from a few of the individuals who have experienced the difference firsthand:

Chronic Pain to a Plan for Recovery: Katelyn's Journey

"I played Division 1 athletics in college, and I have been struggling with my health (knees/back/hips) for the last few years, but more specifically since March with an incident of a compressed right kneecap. Since moving to Chicago and working with Dr. Fisher & his team for the last month, I finally feel that I have a plan towards a full recovery and have noticed significant change.

Dr. Fisher creates a specific plan for your health, and his practice is much more than chiropractic care. Things I have been doing for the last few weeks: laser, physical therapy, chiropractic care, & pain point therapy.

I highly recommend coming into this practice if you are in chronic pain or looking to recover from an injury. Finally on the up and up!"

From Pain to Renewed Mobility - Myriam's Experience at Innovative Nerve & Joint Centers

"Dr. Fisher and staff are amazing! The office is clean and everyone is so friendly! I came in with back, neck, and knee pain. Within days of Dr. Fisher treating me, I noticed a difference. I really do feel 10 years younger! I have more mobility in the areas that I stated earlier. I would recommend any and everyone to come see for yourself!"

From Constant Headaches to Lasting Relief: Ros's Success Story

"I went to Dr. Fisher hoping to get relief from chronic headaches as well as advice on what to do about a recent knee injury. I was not disappointed in either of these areas. I have gone from having headaches several times a week to only a few times each month, which is something I never thought I would be able to say. And when the knee injury required surgery, Dr. Fisher was able to not only set me up with an orthopedic surgeon, but also provide the physical therapy afterward."

These stories represent more than just pain relief. They're about reclaiming daily activities, pursuing passions, and feeling genuinely cared for throughout the process. If you're ready to create your own success story, the FREEDOM Protocol can be your starting point.

Beyond Symptom Relief: The Holistic Advantage

The FREEDOM Protocol understands that your knees don't exist in isolation. Your body is an interconnected masterpiece, where issues in one area can ripple out and affect others. This is why we take a whole-body approach to healing. Let's see how this benefits you:

- **Optimized Treatment: The Whole-Picture Solution**

Maybe that nagging knee pain started after tweaking your ankle a few months ago. Or perhaps a tight hip is unknowingly putting extra strain on your knee. The FREEDOM program looks beyond the obvious. By addressing the entire system and not just the immediate pain point, we tackle the true root of your discomfort. This leads to faster, more sustainable results.

- **Prevention is Key: Strength Beyond the Knee**

Treating your knee is important, but what about protecting it for the future? By strengthening the muscles supporting your knees, hips, and core, and identifying movement patterns that may be causing stress, we create a shield of resilience around your knees. This minimizes the risk of future injuries and flare-ups.

- **Empowered Health: Knowledge is Power**

Imagine understanding why your knee hurts and what you can do about it. The FREEDOM Protocol isn't just about us fixing you. It's about teaching you how your body works and how to make choices that support your knee health over the long term. You become an active partner in your healing journey, which leads to lasting control, not just temporary relief.

Think of it like this: Treating ONLY your knee is like patching a leaky roof without finding the source of the damage. The FREEDOM Protocol helps you address the leak AND reinforce the entire structure for a home (and a body!) that withstands the storms.

Shift Your Mindset: Knee Pain Isn't the Enemy

Knee pain—just those two words can be frustrating and limiting. But what if we shifted the conversation? What if knee pain wasn't the enemy but a messenger trying to tell you something important?

Think of your knee pain as your body's communication, not a life sentence. It's the same with your car: a warning light on your dashboard doesn't mean everything is broken, but it does mean that something needs attention. By understanding what message your knee is sending, you will be able to take steps to fix the underlying issue and prevent it from getting worse.

Don't ignore that twinge or ache in your knee—early intervention is critical to a faster, smoother recovery. The earlier one deals with the problem, the better the chances of preventing complications and getting back to things he or she enjoys doing.

The FREEDOM Protocol has nothing to do with putting band-aids or masking the pain with short-term solutions. We find the root cause and put a plan in place for long-lasting relief. This will assist in giving you the tools and knowledge that will help keep your knees healthy throughout the years.

When you know why your knee pain is occurring, you are brought back into the driver's seat regarding your health. Knowledge allows one to make choices that are thought through about activity levels, exercise, and general lifestyle. You move from being a victim of your body to an active participant in your healing journey.

Analyze to Find the Root Cause

Imagine knee pain is a crime scene. While the first part of a visit is referred to as a "History", our goal is goal is to be a good historian but a better detective. Finding the culprit and achieving lasting relief requires expert investigation. The "Analyze" phase of the FREEDOM Protocol is where we roll up our sleeves and get to the bottom of your pain. Here's how the investigation unfolds.

Analysis Decoded

The first step in solving the puzzle of your knee pain is gathering clues. And you, the patient, are the best source of information! During your initial consultation, we'll take the time to truly understand your "knee story."

Think of this conversation as a collaborative interview. You're the expert on your own body, and we're here to listen closely. We'll ask a series of questions, not just to fill out a form, but to gain insights that point us toward the root cause of your pain. Here are some things we might want to know:

- **Pain Location: Be Specific:** "Inside my knee" is a start, but can you pinpoint it even more? Is it near the front, the back, or the sides? Does the pain feel deep or closer to the surface?
- **Sound Effects:** Does your knee make any strange noises when you move it? Clicking, popping, or grinding sensations can offer valuable clues about what might be going on inside.
- **Triggers and Tamers:** What activities consistently make your knee pain worse? What, if anything, helps alleviate it? Understanding these patterns helps us narrow down potential causes.
- **The Injury Files:** Even those old sprains or seemingly minor incidents matter. Sometimes, seemingly unrelated past injuries can have lingering effects on your knee's health.

This detailed discussion isn't just about checking boxes. It paints a picture of your unique situation. Did the pain start suddenly or sneak up on you? Are you super active at work, or is your lifestyle more sedentary? These and other details help us personalize your analysis and build the most effective treatment plan for YOU so you can reach YOUR GOALS.

Don't be afraid to share everything you think might be relevant. The more complete the picture we have, the better equipped we are to help you find lasting relief.

The Case of the Hidden Issue

Once we have a clearer picture of your knee pain history, it's time for a hands-on examination. Think of this less like a medical test and more like a detective carefully examining a crime scene. Our goal is to uncover clues about how your knee is functioning and what might be causing your discomfort. Here's what you can expect:

- **Movement Matters:** We'll start by gently guiding your knee through its range of motion - bending, straightening, and maybe even a little rotation. This helps us assess any limitations or areas where your movement feels restricted.

- **Stability Check:** Next, we'll test the stability of your knee's various ligaments by applying light pressure in different directions. This allows us to check for any unusual looseness or instability that might be contributing to your pain.

- **Pinpointing the Pain:** We'll carefully check for swelling and any spots that are particularly tender to the touch. Where exactly it hurts helps us determine which structures in your knee might be irritated or injured.

- **Muscle Power:** Often, knee pain is linked to weakness in surrounding muscles. We may test the strength of specific muscle groups around your knee, hips, and core to see if they're providing your knee with the support it needs.

- **Muscle Over Activity:** When a joint is damaged or unstable your body's natural reaction is to protect it. In the short term, absolutely. But is this doesn't resolve it creates long term problems. To add a wrinkle, the damaged joint may not even be your knee. An injured ankle that "doesn't hurt" can cause problems in knee. Where there's pain isn't always where the problem is.

This exam is designed to be informative, not painful. We'll work together to understand how your knee reacts to different movements and pressures. Open communication is key – let us know if anything feels uncomfortable, and we'll adjust accordingly.

Remember, these physical tests are just another way we gather evidence to crack the case of your knee pain. The insights gained here, combined with your history, help us paint a clearer picture of what's going on and how to best get you back on track.

Behind the Scenes: When Imaging Sheds Light

Sometimes, to truly understand what's happening inside your knee, we need a visual. Think of imaging techniques like high-powered flashlights, allowing us to illuminate areas that can't be seen with the naked eye. Here's what these tools can reveal:

- **X-rays:** The Bone Detectives X-rays are excellent for examining bones. They can show us fractures, arthritis, or other changes in bone structure that might be contributing to your pain.
- **Ultrasounds & MRIs:** Seeing the Soft Stuff These technologies let us visualize soft tissues like cartilage, ligaments, tendons, and muscles.

This helps detect tears, inflammation, or degeneration – all of which can be major players in knee pain.

We don't order imaging for every patient. But in some cases, it provides that "Aha!" moment, confirming a diagnosis or revealing a problem we wouldn't have found otherwise.

While your history and physical exam are crucial, imaging can provide that missing puzzle piece. It might confirm what we suspect, or surprise us with a hidden factor leading to your pain. When used strategically, imaging is an invaluable tool that helps us create the most effective treatment plan possible.

Diagnosis: Your Roadmap to Relief

Imagine trying to navigate a new city without a map – chances are you'd get lost, frustrated, and spend a lot of time wandering down the wrong streets. Trying to treat knee pain without a precise diagnosis is just as confusing. Without knowing the exact cause of your discomfort, it's easy to waste time on ineffective treatments. An accurate diagnosis eliminates guesswork and focuses your efforts on solutions that will actually work. It's the difference between throwing darts at a target you can't see and hitting the bullseye every time.

When you receive a diagnosis, something like a torn meniscus or the beginnings of osteoarthritis, it changes everything. No longer are you simply suffering from "knee pain." You gain a clear understanding of what's going on inside your joint – and understanding is power. You can make informed choices about your treatment, ask the right questions, and feel like you have some control over your recovery.

More importantly, an accurate diagnosis has enormous preventative benefits. Knowing the root cause of your knee pain can highlight areas of weakness or imbalance that might be putting you at risk of further injury. With this knowledge, we can develop a plan to strengthen those areas and help you prevent future problems, keeping your knees healthy and pain-free for many years to come.

Think of an accurate diagnosis as the crucial starting point on your recovery journey. It reveals your destination and the best route to get there. It allows for highly targeted treatment, empowers you with essential knowledge, and lays the foundation for long-lasting knee health.

Your Knee Health Exam: The Essentials

Ready to unleash the detective within and uncover the culprit behind your knee pain? Here at the FREEDOM

Protocol, we believe in a collaborative approach. This checklist outlines what you can generally expect during a thorough knee health evaluation, but remember, this is YOUR journey. Don't hesitate to ask questions, share any concerns, and be an active participant in the process.

The Pre-Game Prep: Gathering the Clues

- Detailed History Discussion: Come prepared to share your medical history, past injuries, lifestyle habits, and anything else you think might be relevant. The more information we have, the better equipped we are to understand your unique case.
- Open Communication is Key: We encourage open and honest communication. Don't downplay pain or hesitate to mention seemingly minor details. Everything you share can be a valuable clue in solving the mystery of your knee pain.

Putting Your Knee to the Test

- Comprehensive Physical Exam: Our chiropractors will perform a series of gentle tests to assess your knee's range of motion, stability, strength, and any areas of tenderness. This hands-on examination allows us to see how your knee functions and identify potential areas of concern.

- Imaging When Needed: X-rays, ultrasounds, or MRIs may be recommended to get a clearer picture of what's happening inside your knee. We'll discuss the potential benefits and answer any questions you might have about imaging technology.

Understanding the Results

- Open Explanation of Your Diagnosis: We'll take the time to explain your diagnosis in clear, understandable language. You'll walk away with a clear understanding of the cause of your pain and the treatment options available.
- Discussing Your Treatment Plan: There's no one-size-fits-all solution at the FREEDOM Protocol. We'll work with you to create a personalized treatment plan tailored to your specific needs and goals. You'll be an active participant in every step of your recovery journey.

This checklist is just a starting point. The FREEDOM Protocol is dedicated to partnering with you to achieve lasting knee health. We'll equip you with the knowledge and tools you need to make informed decisions about your care and feel empowered to live an active life, free from knee pain.

So, are you ready to become a knee health detective? Let's get started on uncovering the cause of your pain and get you back to the activities you love!

Cutting Edge Techniques in Action

Advanced Tools for Relief

You've heard of traditional treatments for knee pain, but in the FREEDOM Protocol, we like to go the extra mile. Let's take a look at a few of the cutting-edge techniques that we use to help you find relief and restore healthy knee function.

Cold Laser Therapy: Not the Lasers from Sci-Fi Movies

Forget the idea of burning lasers! Think of this as a gentle boost for your body's own healing abilities. Cold laser therapy uses a specific type of light that's able to reach those deep knee tissues. As a result, it can help manage inflammation, ease pain, improve blood flow, and encourage your body to repair itself faster. It's a totally painless and relaxing way to tackle what's causing your discomfort.

Trigenics®: Retraining Your Muscles

Think of Trigenics® as a way to reprogram the way your knee works. Our chiropractors are specially trained to analyze those tiny signals between your brain, nerves, and the muscles around your knee. Sometimes, those signals get a bit scrambled, and that causes pain. Trigenics® helps fix the communication mix-up so your knee can start moving with ease again.

Infrared Therapy: Soothing Warmth with a Purpose

This treatment uses a special type of light that sends a warm, soothing feeling deep into your knee joint. It helps increase blood flow (always a good thing when it comes to healing!), reduces inflammation, and encourages your tissues to rebuild. Sometimes we'll combine it with other therapies to maximize how great your knees can feel.

Movement Therapy: Not Just Random Exercises

It's not about "just do this exercise" – movement therapy is way more personalized. We focus on pinpointing those muscles around your knee that might be weak, too tight, or just not coordinated quite right. Our chiropractors create a plan to address your specific needs, so you can regain strength, flexibility, and smooth, pain-free movement.

With the FREEDOM Protocol, it's not just about masking the pain. Our goal is to help you understand what's happening with your knees, treat the underlying problems, and teach you ways to keep your knees strong and healthy for the long haul!

Softwave Therapy

The damage to your knee may have been there for months, or even years. We need to not only restore normal function but also help your body repair the damage. Nicknamed "the stem cell machine", softwave therapy works to recruit stem cells to the treatment area to fast track healing in areas where the body hasn't been able to heal on its own.

The Power of Combining Techniques

The true strength of the FREEDOM Protocol lies in strategically combining these techniques. It's NOT about a one-and-done approach. It's about expert analysis to identify your individual needs and create a comprehensive plan, using the full range of tools in our arsenal to get you back to your active life.

Success Stories

The true power of the FREEDOM Protocol lies in its ability to transform lives. Let's take a look at two individuals who found relief and regained their active lifestyles:

- **Maggie the Runner: Back on the Marathon Trail**

Constant knee pain threatened to sideline Maggie, a dedicated marathoner, for good. Through targeted mobilization techniques and deep soft tissue work, we addressed chronic muscular imbalances that were creating stress on her knees. Additionally, gait analysis revealed a subtle flaw in her running form. By retraining her running patterns, we helped her body move more efficiently, reducing stress on her knees. Maggie is now back to training for marathons, pain-free.

- **Grandpa Joe: Stability is Key**

For Joe, knee pain made even simple tasks like walking his dog a struggle. His FREEDOM Protocol treatment focused on building the core and leg strength needed to improve the stability of his knees. With a personalized exercise program, he gradually but steadily rebuilt the support his knees lacked. Now, he's enjoying long walks with his furry companion and has enough energy to keep up with his grandkids.

These success stories illustrate how the FREEDOM Protocol addresses more than just the symptoms of knee pain. By identifying and treating the root causes, we empower individuals to not only find relief but also reclaim the activities they love.

The Benefits of Innovation

Investing in cutting-edge techniques for knee care offers a wealth of benefits for patients. Firstly, these advanced approaches often speed up your recovery time. This means you'll experience the relief you're seeking much sooner compared to relying on more traditional, passive treatments.

Secondly, these techniques focus on addressing the root cause of your knee pain, not just masking the symptoms. This translates to a more complete and sustainable recovery, maximizing your chances of staying pain-free for the long term.

Finally, because cutting-edge techniques can be precisely targeted to your specific diagnosis and individual needs, they tend to be far more effective than a generic, one-size-fits-all approach. This personalized element means you're getting the right kind of treatment to optimize your outcome and get you back to being active as quickly as possible.

Implementing New Techniques

When discussing cutting-edge techniques for your knee care, it's important to be an active participant in the process. Do some research and ask your healthcare provider specific questions about the recommended techniques and how they might help you. Open communication is key here – it's perfectly fine to express any concerns or preferences you may have, as not every technique is suitable for everyone.

Remember, the best results often come when cutting-edge techniques are combined with your own active participation in the recovery process. Your commitment to things like at-home exercises greatly amplifies the effectiveness of the treatments you receive in the clinic.

The FREEDOM Protocol is dedicated to offering the latest advancements while prioritizing your individual needs and comfort. Our goal is to help you move beyond pain and into a healthier, more active future.

Treatment for Mobility

Mobility: Your Knees' Best Friend

The FREEDOM Protocol views mobility-focused treatment as a powerful tool for achieving lasting knee health. This approach goes beyond traditional treatments that focus solely on the knee itself. Through specialized manual therapies like joint mobilizations, targeted soft tissue techniques to release tight muscles, and carefully designed functional exercises, we help your body move more efficiently, reducing stress on your knees and unlocking your full potential for pain-free activity.

It's important to understand that mobility isn't just about flexibility. While stretching can be helpful, true mobility-focused treatment looks at the bigger picture. It's about identifying and addressing restrictions throughout your body that might be subtly affecting your alignment and movement patterns. Our goal is to help you retrain how you move, so your body works with you, not against you, protecting your knees from both current pain and future injuries.

Beyond Static Stretches

The traditional approach to knee pain often involves static treatments like rest, ice, compression, and elevation (RICE), as well as pain medication and anti-inflammatory drugs. While these methods can offer temporary relief, they often fall short in addressing the root cause of the problem. They tend to focus on reducing inflammation and pain but neglect the underlying issues that may be contributing to the discomfort, such as muscle imbalances, joint restrictions, or movement dysfunction.

Mobility-focused treatment, on the other hand, takes a more proactive and holistic approach. It recognizes that knee pain is often a symptom of a broader issue, and that restoring proper movement patterns is key to long-term relief. This approach involves a combination of:

- **Manual Therapy:** Hands-on techniques like joint mobilizations and soft tissue work to improve joint range of motion and release muscle tightness.
- **Targeted Exercises:** Specific exercises designed to strengthen weak muscles, improve flexibility, and retrain movement patterns.
- **Patient Education:** Empowering patients with knowledge about their bodies and how to move correctly to avoid further injury.

By addressing the root cause of the problem and restoring optimal movement, mobility-focused treatment offers several advantages over traditional static treatments:

- **Long-Term Relief**: Instead of just masking the pain, mobility treatment aims to correct the underlying issues, leading to more sustainable and lasting relief.
- **Improved Function**: By restoring proper movement patterns, mobility treatment can enhance your knee's function, allowing you to move more freely and easily.
- **Reduced Risk of Re-Injury**: By addressing muscle imbalances and movement dysfunction, mobility treatment can help prevent future injuries and keep your knees healthy in the long run.
- **Enhanced Performance**: For athletes and active individuals, improved mobility can lead to better performance and reduced risk of injury during sports and activities.

If you're struggling with knee pain, don't settle for temporary fixes. Explore the benefits of mobility-focused treatment and discover a path towards lasting relief and improved function.

ACTION STEP: Get Your Knee Pain Relief Handbook. Master 9 Key Stretches from Home To Eliminate Knee Pain.

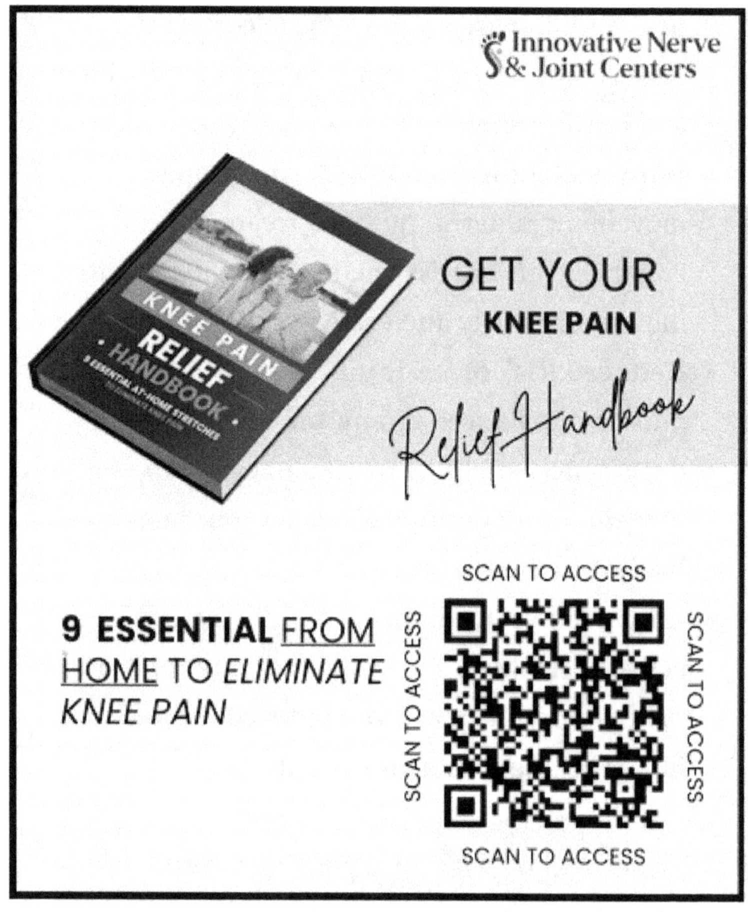

Unlock Your Path To Knee Pain Relief Now: Call (833) 359-6099 To Speak With An Expert Today!

3

———

DEBUNKING ALTERNATIVES

Bill shuffled into my office, his shoulders slumped, a weary expression etched on his face. He clutched a thick manila folder overflowing with medical records, a testament to his years-long battle with debilitating knee pain. "I've tried it all, Doc," he sighed, "painkillers, injections, even physical therapy. Nothing seems to work. My surgeon says my only option now is a knee replacement, but I'm just not ready for that." Bill, a retired carpenter, longed to return to his woodworking hobby and keep up with his energetic grandchildren, but his knee pain had become a constant roadblock. He'd resigned himself to a life of limitations, believing surgery was his inevitable fate.

We discussed the FREEDOM Protocol, explaining our focus on identifying and addressing the underlying causes of knee pain, not just masking the symptoms. Bill, though initially skeptical, agreed to give it a try. His assessment revealed significant weakness in his hip and core muscles, contributing to instability and poor knee alignment. We developed a personalized plan, incorporating targeted exercises, manual therapy, and cold laser therapy to reduce inflammation and improve joint function.

A few months later, a different Bill walked into my office. The weariness was gone, replaced by a renewed sense of vitality. He held a small, intricately carved wooden bird, a testament to his rediscovered passion. "I can't thank you enough, Dr. Fisher," he said, a genuine smile lighting up his face. "I'm back in my workshop, and I can even keep up with the grandkids again. This program has given me back my life."

Individual results may vary.

Bill's story highlights a crucial point: while conventional approaches like medication and surgery can be necessary in certain cases, they often fall short in addressing the root cause of knee pain. The focus on quick fixes can sometimes overshadow the potential for true, lasting healing.

Limitations of Conventional Medicine

When knee pain strikes, the default course of action often involves medication, injections, or in severe cases, surgery. While these conventional approaches can offer temporary relief in some cases, they frequently fail to address the root cause of the problem, leading to a frustrating cycle of recurring pain.

Medication & Surgery: The Limits

If you're frustrated with limited success when managing knee pain, it's important to understand why these common approaches might fall short. Think about pain medication – whether over-the-counter or prescription-strength. While it might offer much-needed temporary relief, it simply numbs the sensation of pain. This means the root cause of your discomfort remains unaddressed. Long-term reliance on medication often becomes an unhealthy cycle and can even lead to unwanted side effects.

Surgery, while necessary for severe cases like major ligament tears or advanced arthritis, isn't a guarantee of lasting pain relief. Even a technically successful surgery won't prevent problems from returning if the underlying reasons that contributed to the damage in the first place aren't addressed. Imagine surgery as a major repair, but if the forces and conditions that caused the damage are still present, future deterioration is possible.

The FREEDOM Protocol believes in exploring alternatives that go beyond simply masking symptoms or offering temporary fixes. Remember, your knee pain is a valuable signal from your body. Our approach is to listen to that signal and find solutions that promote true healing and lasting knee health.

Beyond Patient Stories: Limited Results

Sarah hoped that arthroscopic knee surgery would be her ticket back to pain-free running. Initially, it was! The relief was amazing, but her joy was short-lived. Within a year, that familiar ache crept back into her knee. It was discouraging, and no one seemed to have answers as to why this happened or how to stop it from happening again.

Joe managed his knee pain for years by taking over-the-counter painkillers. They made his daily life bearable, but bearable was a far cry from the active life he longed for. The medication dulled the pain enough to get through work, but hiking trips with his family or playing ball with the grandkids were always a struggle. He knew there had to be a better way to manage his knee pain, a way that didn't just make it tolerable but truly made it better.

These stories aren't unique. Many people experience the disappointment of treatments that offer temporary relief or only partially address the problem. This frustration is often what leads them to seek alternative solutions like the FREEDOM Protocol.

Holistic Healing: A Wider View

The FREEDOM method understands that your knee pain isn't just about discomfort, it's a message your body is trying to send. Instead of simply throwing painkillers at the problem or assuming surgery is the only solution, we take a wider view. Our holistic approach focuses on three crucial aspects:

First, we play detective. We look beyond the immediate pain in your knee, understanding that the true cause might lie elsewhere. Maybe a past ankle sprain is still affecting your alignment, or weak hip muscles are throwing off your gait and creating extra stress on your knees. Getting to the root of the issue is the only way to unlock a lasting solution.

Second, we don't believe in temporary fixes. Our goal is to address the actual cause of your discomfort, making today better and minimizing the chances of your pain coming back down the line.

Finally, we believe in empowering you. No one should feel forever dependent on medications or worry their knee will keep them from doing what they love. We want to give you the knowledge, exercises, and everyday habits that let you play an active role in your recovery process and maintain healthy knees for years to come.

Think of this holistic approach as providing your body with the tools it needs to heal itself. It's also about giving you the guidance and support to feel confident in taking charge of your own health.

Questions for Your Doctor: Seeking Alternatives

If you feel stuck in a cycle of knee pain that isn't fully improving with conventional treatments, don't be afraid to advocate for yourself. Open communication with your healthcare provider is crucial. Here are some questions to consider asking:

- What do you believe is at the root of my knee pain? *Don't settle for a vague "wear and tear" answer. Ask them to explain the specific factors they believe are contributing to your discomfort.*
- Are there alternative or complementary therapies, in addition to what we're already doing, that might be helpful in my case? *This shows you're open to exploring different options.*

- What can I actively do to prevent this pain from coming back or getting worse? *This emphasizes your desire to be a proactive participant in your health.*

It's perfectly okay to seek a second opinion or explore different approaches if you aren't getting the results you need. FREEDOM is dedicated to offering a fresh perspective, empowering you with knowledge, and designing a personalized treatment plan to get you back to living an active, pain-free life.

The Myth of Quick Fixes

The Quick Fix Trap

When you're dealing with knee pain, every day can feel like a struggle. The constant discomfort can make even the simplest tasks an uphill battle. It's understandable to want the pain to just STOP – and want it to stop NOW. This desperation is why the promise of "quick fixes" holds such strong appeal. The idea of a pill, an injection, or a surgical procedure that could magically erase the pain is incredibly tempting. Unfortunately, these solutions often trade instant gratification for lasting relief.

Temporary Relief, Lasting Problems

Sometimes the limitations of quick fixes become clear through shared experiences. Let's take a look at Maggie and Bill:

- **Maggie's Cortisone Cycle:** Chronic tendonitis plagued Maggie, making her favorite activities miserable. Cortisone injections would magically erase the pain for a few weeks, but then it always crept back. Each flare-up seemed worse than the last. She realized these injections were simply masking a deeper problem that wasn't being addressed.
- **Bill's Surgery Setback:** Bill had knee surgery to repair a torn meniscus. The surgery itself was successful, and the initial rehab went well. However, despite his efforts, he never quite regained the same strength or stability in his knee. Months later, that familiar ache returned. This left Bill feeling defeated and wondering what other options even existed.

These stories illustrate how a focus on immediate relief can sometimes overshadow the need for a long-term solution. The FREEDOM Program believes it's important to look beyond the quick fix and focus on achieving the kind of healing that lasts.

Invest in Lasting Health

It's important to be aware of the potential pitfalls when seeking knee pain relief. Be wary of any treatment that promises instant results without addressing the underlying cause of your problem. While the idea of immediate relief is appealing, these quick fixes rarely offer a lasting solution.

Ask questions! Consult with your healthcare provider about the long-term consequences of treatments focused solely on temporarily easing your pain. Be an advocate for your own health and seek providers who share your desire for a sustainable solution. True healing takes time and effort, but the payoff is lasting relief and freedom from the cycle of recurring pain.

The FREEDOM Program is dedicated to helping you avoid the allure of quick fixes and embrace the potential of lasting knee health. We're committed to personalized treatment plans that focus on addressing the root of your pain, offering you a path toward true healing without the need for constant short-term fixes.

Beyond the Band-Aid: Escape the Cycle

Don't underestimate the power of being an active participant in your knee health journey. Here are some crucial ways to avoid getting stuck in a cycle of temporary solutions:

- **Ask Questions:** Your healthcare provider is a valuable partner in your healing. Don't hesitate to ask questions like, "Will this treatment address the cause of my pain or just mask it?" and "What are the potential long-term benefits and risks of this approach?"

- **Seek a Holistic Approach:** Look for providers who aren't content with simply putting a temporary band-aid on your knee pain. The right practitioner will prioritize uncovering the 'why' behind your discomfort and create a treatment plan that creates a foundation for lasting relief.

- **Be Patient & Consistent:** Quick fixes might make big promises, but true healing often requires a slower, steadier approach. Don't be discouraged if the results aren't immediate. Commit to a treatment plan that focuses on sustainable solutions, and trust that consistency with things like exercises and recommended lifestyle changes will pay off in the long run.

Taking charge of your knee health means seeking out solutions with your long-term well-being at the forefront.

FREEDOM is committed to helping you break free from the cycle of quick fixes. We prioritize a long-term approach that not only relieves your current pain but also empowers you to enjoy an active life without the fear of recurring knee problems.

Overlooked Aspects of Knee Health

The Power of Lifestyle

While knee pain might make you think primarily of surgeries and medication, it's important to realize the profound impact your daily life has on your joints. Your nutrition, your posture, even your level of stress – these seemingly unrelated factors can significantly influence your knee health.

Think of your body as a finely tuned system. When you provide it with the fuel and support it needs, it has a remarkable ability to heal and protect itself. This includes your knees! By making small, positive changes in your daily habits, you can tap into this natural healing potential and minimize the everyday stressors that contribute to knee pain. While it's not always the only solution, a focus on lifestyle can be a powerful complement to any knee treatment plan.

Small Changes, Big Impact

Small changes can truly have a powerful impact on knee health. It's amazing how seemingly simple lifestyle shifts can make a huge difference for those suffering from knee pain. Let's look at a few examples.

Mary's Anti-Inflammatory Switch: Mary battled with chronic knee pain, trying medication, physical therapy, and even injections with limited relief. Finally, she discovered that chronic inflammation was a significant factor behind her discomfort. Her diet, full of processed foods and sugary treats, was keeping her body in a state of constant inflammation. By switching to whole, anti-inflammatory foods, Mary's knees, and her overall health, saw a dramatic improvement.

Mike's Posture Fix: Mike assumed his knee pain was just something he had to put up with as he aged. However, a dedicated physical therapist helped him realize that his posture was having a major impact on his joints. With simple adjustments to how he stood, lifted objects, and even how he walked, Mike felt a remarkable reduction in his knee pain and found new strength and energy.

Lisa's Shoe Swap: Lisa, an avid runner, ignored her mild knee discomfort for months. It wasn't until a running coach suggested she try a different type of shoe that she found relief. Her old shoes offered minimal support, leading to poor alignment and extra strain on her knees. The right pair of shoes made all the difference, allowing her to pursue her passion for running pain-free.

These stories illustrate that lasting knee health isn't always about major interventions. Often, small but strategic changes in your daily life can yield impressive results!

Hidden Costs of Ignoring Knee Health

Ignoring the impact of nutrition, posture, and lifestyle on your knees can shortchange your body's healing process. If issues like inflammation, poor ergonomics, or chronic stress are contributing to your knee pain, relying solely on quick-fix treatments might only provide temporary relief. This could potentially trap you in a cycle where the true cause of your pain goes unaddressed.

Additionally, choosing to live with untreated chronic knee pain can significantly impact your quality of life. Over time, it may limit your activity levels, leading to other health concerns, or negatively affect your overall well-being.

The FREEDOM Program believes in proactive care. We'll help you identify how lifestyle factors are affecting your knees and create a personalized plan for sustainable change. This holistic approach maximizes your healing potential, offering you lasting pain relief and increased resilience.

Knee-Friendly Daily Habits

The wonderful thing about focusing on lifestyle changes is that it puts you back in control! Small, consistent choices made each day can pave the way to healthier, happier knees. Here are some key areas of focus:

- **Nutrition:** Make whole foods the stars of the show. Fill your plate with lots of colorful fruits and vegetables. These powerhouses provide nutrients that naturally fight inflammation. Limit processed foods, as these can contribute to the kind of inflammation that aggravates joint pain.
- **Movement:** Be mindful of your body. Simple posture awareness throughout the day, like standing taller or adjusting how you lift things, can protect your knees from unnecessary strain.

- **Stress Management:** Stress can manifest as physical tension and worsening pain. Find healthy ways to manage stress, whether it's calming meditation, deep breathing, or spending time outdoors.
- **Rest and Recovery:** Your body heals while you rest. Prioritize quality sleep and build downtime into your schedule, especially after periods of increased activity.
- **Maintaining a healthy weight:** This isn't a comfortable conversation but it's important to have. Every extra pound you have puts an extra four pounds of stress on your body.

The FREEDOM Protocol views your health as a holistic, interconnected system. We'll work with you to identify the lifestyle factors that might be impacting your knees and help you create sustainable habits for lasting improvement.

Why FREEDOM Works Where Others Fail

Beyond the Standard Approach

If you've tried standard knee pain treatments but still feel stuck in a cycle of pain and limitations, it's time to explore something different. FREEDOM breaks the mold of conventional care, prioritizing a personalized and empowering approach.

Instead of simply offering quick fixes that only mask the pain, we get curious. We thoroughly analyze your history, your movement patterns, and all the unique factors that contribute to YOUR knee discomfort. Once we understand the "why" behind the pain, we can create a treatment plan that truly addresses the root of the problem.

Our approach is holistic because we know your knee doesn't exist in isolation. Everything from an old ankle sprain to weak core muscles can increase stress on your knees. We take the time to identify these weaknesses and imbalances. This ensures you get the comprehensive support needed for true healing and lasting pain relief.

The FREEDOM Protocol believes in giving you back control. We don't just treat your knee; we teach you about your body. You'll learn why the pain started, how to change everyday habits that might be adding strain, and how to be proactive about protecting your knees for years to come. This knowledge is a powerful tool, allowing you to feel confident about managing your knee health and reclaiming the active lifestyle you deserve!

Passive vs. Active: A New Approach

While finding relief from your current knee pain is likely your top priority, FREEDOM offers benefits that extend far beyond simply feeling better in the moment. Our approach is designed to empower you with lasting improvements in your knee health. Here's what you can expect:

- **Reduced Pain & Improved Function**: Pain might be what brings you in the door, but the results shouldn't stop there. We'll work with you to reduce discomfort and restore your ability to do what matters to you. Whether it's a pain-free walk with your dog, playing with your grandkids, or returning to your favorite way of exercising, we'll help you reach those goals.
- **Increased Strength and Resilience**: Knee pain is often a symptom of underlying weaknesses and imbalances. Our approach builds strength in the right places, making your knees more adaptable to the twists, turns, and unexpected stresses that life throws at them.
- **Prevention of Future Problems**: By addressing the root cause of your knee pain and equipping you with personalized strategies, we help set

the stage for lasting results. This reduced risk of recurring pain translates to fewer frustrations and limitations down the road.

- **Peace of Mind:** Knee pain can make you feel vulnerable and uncertain about the future. The FREEDOM Protocol replaces that worry with knowledge and tools. You'll understand your body better and feel confident in your ability to protect your knees and enjoy an active life without the fear of pain holding you back.

These benefits create a ripple effect, positively impacting your overall well-being and allowing you to live life on your terms!

The Power of Proactive Healing

The FREEDOM Program isn't about a set of quick fixes to make your pain magically disappear. It's about embracing a deeper, more empowered approach to your knee health. This requires a mindset shift, one that emphasizes open investigation, consistency, and patience.

We encourage you to be curious about potential causes of your knee pain that you might not have considered. Sometimes it's not just about the knee itself, but how your whole body moves and its hidden weak links.

Understanding these interconnected factors is crucial for finding solutions that truly work for you.

Think of your treatment plan, whether it's exercises or lifestyle adjustments, as essential, non-negotiable investments in your future. While it's easy to get lured by quick fixes, those only offer a fleeting illusion of relief. Consistency is what builds healthier, more resilient knees and paves the way to lasting improvement.

Finally, remember that healing takes time, especially when dealing with chronic knee pain. Trust the individualized plan we develop for you. Celebrate even small victories along the way – these wins build confidence and motivation.

Are you ready to ditch the cycle of knee pain and become an active participant in shaping a healthier future? The FREEDOM Protocol is here to partner with you on this empowering journey.

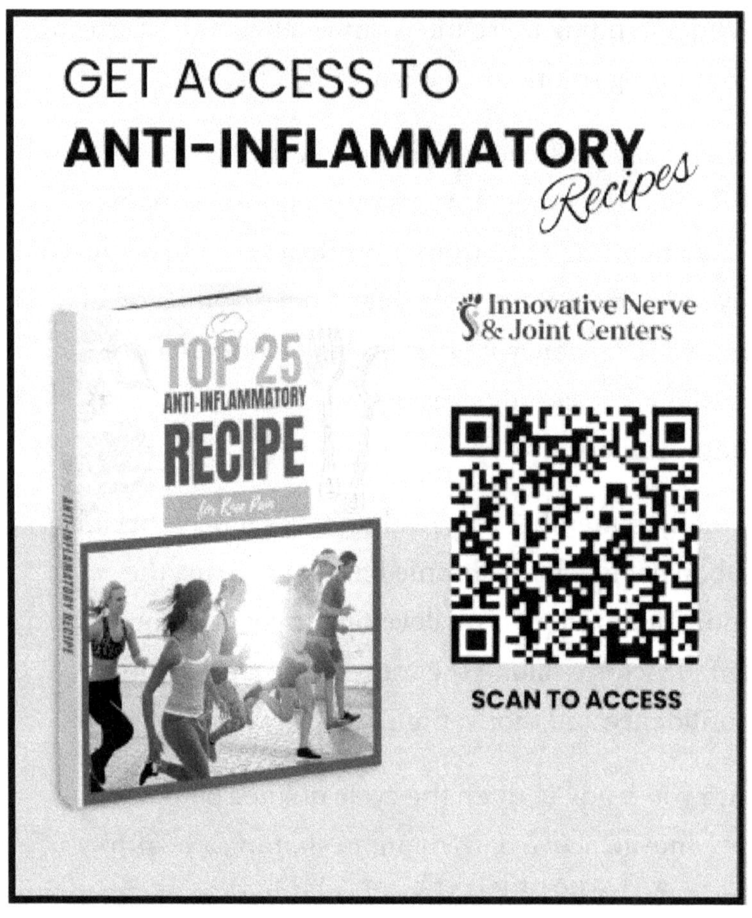

Unlock Your Path To Knee Pain Relief Now: Call (833) 359-6099 To Speak With An Expert Today!

4

———

MAINTAINING KNEE HEALTH
AT WORK

Ana, a graphic designer, sat across from me, her brow furrowed in frustration. "My knee pain is making it impossible to focus at work," she explained. "I spend hours hunched over my computer, and by the end of the day, my knees are throbbing. I've tried standing desks, ergonomic chairs, everything! Nothing seems to make a difference." Her story was all too familiar – the demands of a desk-bound job taking a toll on her body. She loved her work, but the constant pain was threatening to derail her career and her active lifestyle outside of the office.

Ana's assessment revealed a combination of factors contributing to her knee pain: tight hip flexors from prolonged sitting, weak core muscles, and poor posture. We implemented the FREEDOM Protocol, focusing on targeted exercises to address these specific issues. We also educated her on the importance of incorporating movement breaks and proper ergonomic setups into her workday.

A few weeks later, Ana returned for a follow-up, a noticeable lightness in her step. "I can't believe how much better I feel!" she exclaimed. "The exercises are actually making a difference. I'm moving more freely, and my knee pain has significantly decreased. I even convinced my boss to get us all standing desk converters!" Ana's enthusiasm was contagious – not only was she experiencing relief, but she was also actively changing her work environment for the better. Her journey serves as a powerful reminder that even small changes can make a big impact. While her success isn't a guarantee for everyone, it offers a glimpse into the possibilities.

Results are not typical. Your experience may vary.

The modern workplace, while offering convenience and connectivity, often presents unique challenges to our physical well-being.

Understanding the Impact of Work on Knee Health

You might not think of your 9-to-5 as a contact sport, but the truth is, our daily work routines can put a surprising amount of wear and tear on our knees. It's not just manual labor jobs that pose a risk; even seemingly harmless activities like sitting at a desk or standing for long periods can gradually contribute to knee pain and dysfunction.

Think about it:

- **Repetitive Movements:** Whether it's typing on a keyboard, operating machinery, or stocking shelves, repetitive movements can strain the tendons and ligaments around your knee joint, leading to inflammation and pain.
- **Prolonged Sitting:** Sitting for hours on end might seem like a restful position, but it actually puts your knees in a vulnerable position. When your knees are bent for extended periods, the cartilage within the joint doesn't receive the nourishment it needs from synovial fluid, which acts as a lubricant. This can lead to stiffness, decreased range of motion, and eventually, pain.
- **Standing for Long Periods:** While standing engages your muscles more than sitting, it can also put excessive pressure on your knees, especially if you have weak muscles or poor posture. This can lead to fatigue, inflammation, and pain in the knee joint.

- **Awkward Postures**: Many work tasks involve bending, twisting, or reaching, which can put your knees in awkward positions and strain the surrounding tissues. Over time, these repetitive strains can lead to chronic pain and dysfunction.

Office Work and the Perils of Prolonged Sitting

Office work, with its emphasis on sitting for extended periods, presents unique challenges for knee health. The sedentary nature of this work environment can lead to several negative consequences:

- **Decreased Joint Lubrication**: When you sit for long periods, your knee joints don't move through their full range of motion. This limits the circulation of synovial fluid, which is essential for nourishing and lubricating the cartilage within the joint. Over time, this can lead to cartilage degeneration and increased friction, contributing to pain and stiffness.
- **Muscle Weakness**: Prolonged sitting can weaken the muscles that support your knee joint, such as your quadriceps and hamstrings. These muscles play a crucial role in stabilizing your knee and absorbing shock during

movement. When they're weak, your knee joint becomes more vulnerable to injury.

- **Poor Circulation:** Sitting for extended periods can also impair blood flow to your legs and knees. This can lead to a buildup of waste products and inflammation, further contributing to pain and stiffness.

Manual Labor and Repetitive Strain Injuries

While office work poses its own set of challenges, manual labor jobs often place a more immediate and intense strain on the knees. The repetitive nature of tasks like heavy lifting, kneeling, squatting, and climbing can lead to overuse injuries and chronic pain.

- **Heavy Lifting:** Improper lifting techniques can put immense stress on the knee joints, especially when combined with heavy loads. This can lead to ligament sprains, meniscus tears, and even damage to the cartilage within the joint.

- **Kneeling and Squatting:** Jobs that require frequent kneeling or squatting can irritate the tendons and bursae (fluid-filled sacs that cushion the joint) around the knee. This can lead to conditions like bursitis (inflammation of the bursae) and tendonitis (inflammation of the tendons).

- **Repetitive Movements:** Tasks that involve repetitive bending, twisting, or climbing can strain the muscles and ligaments around the knee, leading to inflammation and pain. Over time, this can contribute to the development of osteoarthritis, a degenerative joint disease.

Industry-Specific Concerns

Different industries present unique challenges for knee health. Let's take a look at a few examples:

- **Construction:** Construction workers often face a combination of heavy lifting, kneeling, squatting, and climbing, putting their knees at high risk of injury. They may also be exposed to harsh weather conditions, which can exacerbate joint pain.
- **Healthcare:** Nurses, aides, and other healthcare professionals spend long hours on their feet, often lifting and moving patients. This can lead to knee pain, fatigue, and overuse injuries.
- **Service Industries:** Workers in restaurants, retail, and other service industries often stand for extended periods, walk long distances, and

perform repetitive tasks like bending and lifting. These activities can strain the knees and contribute to pain and discomfort.

- **Agriculture:** Agricultural workers engage in physically demanding tasks like planting, harvesting, and caring for livestock. These activities often involve kneeling, squatting, and lifting heavy objects, putting significant stress on the knees.

Whether you're a desk jockey or a manual laborer, the demands of your work can silently chip away at your knee health. The good news is that understanding these risks is the first step towards protecting your knees. By recognizing the hidden strains of daily tasks and the specific challenges of your profession, you can take proactive measures to safeguard your joints and maintain a lifetime of pain-free movement. Remember, your knees are resilient, but they need your care and attention to thrive in the workplace.

Ergonomic Solutions for a Healthier Workplace

Transforming your workspace into a knee-friendly zone doesn't require a major overhaul. Simple adjustments to your setup can make a world of difference in reducing strain and promoting long-term knee health.

Let's dive into the key elements of an ergonomic office setup:

- **Optimal Chair and Desk Setup:** Your chair should be adjusted so that your feet rest flat on the floor, with your knees bent at a comfortable 90-degree angle. Your backrest should provide adequate lumbar support, maintaining the natural curve of your spine. Armrests should allow your shoulders to relax and your elbows to rest at a comfortable angle, typically close to your body.

- **The Importance of a Standing Desk:** Prolonged sitting is a major culprit in knee pain. A standing desk allows you to alternate between sitting and standing throughout the day, reducing the sustained pressure on your knees. This can improve circulation, engage your muscles, and alleviate stiffness. If a full standing desk isn't feasible, consider a standing desk converter that sits on top of your existing desk.

- **Footrests and Their Benefits:** If your feet don't comfortably reach the floor when sitting, a footrest can provide much-needed support. It helps maintain proper posture, reduces strain on your lower back and knees, and promotes better circulation in your legs.

- **Keyboard and Mouse Positioning:** Your keyboard and mouse should be positioned so that your wrists are straight and your forearms are parallel to the floor. This neutral position minimizes strain on your wrists, elbows, and shoulders, which can indirectly affect your knee alignment and function. Avoid reaching or extending your arms excessively, as this can create tension and contribute to poor posture.

Manual Labor Ergonomics: Protecting Your Knees on the Job

If your work involves manual labor, you're no stranger to the physical demands it places on your body, especially your knees. But with the right approach, you can minimize the risk of injury and keep your knees healthy for years to come. Let's explore some essential ergonomic strategies:

- **Proper Lifting Techniques:** Lifting heavy objects incorrectly can wreak havoc on your knees. Instead of relying on your back, bend at your hips and knees, keeping your back straight. Hold the object close to your body and avoid twisting motions as you lift. If an object is too heavy, don't hesitate to ask for help or use a mechanical aid.

- **Using Assistive Devices:** Dollies, carts, hand trucks, and other assistive devices are your allies in the workplace. They can significantly reduce the load on your knees by allowing you to roll or push heavy objects instead of carrying them. Whenever possible, utilize these tools to minimize strain on your joints.

- **Protective Gear:** If your job involves frequent kneeling or squatting, wearing knee pads can provide valuable cushioning and support. Knee braces can also offer additional stability and protection for those with pre-existing knee conditions or a history of injury.

- **Taking Breaks and Stretching:** Don't underestimate the power of rest and movement. Incorporate regular breaks into your workday to give your knees a chance to rest and recover. Use these breaks to perform simple stretches that target your quads, hamstrings, and calves. This can help prevent muscle fatigue, improve flexibility, and reduce the risk of injury.

By implementing these ergonomic principles, you're not just making your workspace more comfortable; you're actively investing in the long-term health of your knees. Even minor adjustments can have a significant impact on reducing strain and preventing pain. So take a moment to assess your work environment and make the necessary changes to create a space that supports your knees and overall well-being. Your body will thank you!

The Power of Movement Breaks

When you're engrossed in work, it's easy to get stuck in one position for hours on end. However, even short bursts of movement can work wonders for your knee health. These "micro-movements" counteract the negative effects of prolonged sitting or repetitive tasks by:

- **Increasing Circulation:** Movement helps pump blood and nutrients to your knees, reducing stiffness and inflammation.
- **Lubricating Joints:** Moving your knees through their range of motion stimulates the production of synovial fluid, which lubricates the joint and nourishes the cartilage.
- **Preventing Muscle Fatigue:** Regular movement breaks prevent your muscles from becoming tight and fatigued, which can strain your knees.

- **Boosting Energy and Focus:** Getting up and moving can increase blood flow to your brain, improving your energy levels and focus.

Simple Exercises for the Workplace

You don't need a gym membership or fancy equipment to incorporate movement breaks into your workday. Here are a few simple exercises you can do right at your desk or in a small space:

- **Chair Squats:** Stand in front of your chair, feet shoulder-width apart. Slowly lower yourself down as if you're going to sit, but hover just above the seat. Engage your core and push back up to standing. Repeat 10-15 times.
- **Calf Raises:** Stand tall and slowly rise up onto your toes, then lower back down. Repeat 15-20 times. You can do this exercise while holding onto your desk or a wall for balance.
- **Knee Extensions:** Sit in your chair with your feet flat on the floor. Extend one leg out straight, hold for a few seconds, then slowly lower it back down. Repeat 10-15 times on each leg.
- **Walking Meetings:** If you have a meeting that doesn't require a computer screen, suggest a walking meeting. This allows you to get some

exercise while still being productive.

- **Hamstring Stretch at Your Desk:** While seated, extend one leg out straight with your heel on the floor. Lean forward from your hips, keeping your back straight, until you feel a gentle stretch in the back of your thigh. Hold for 30 seconds and repeat on the other side.

- **Seated Hip Flexor Stretch:** Sit on the edge of your chair and bring one knee towards your chest, holding it with both hands. Gently pull your knee closer to your chest until you feel a stretch in the front of your hip. Hold for 30 seconds and repeat on the other side.

- **Ankle Pumps:** While seated or standing, point your toes and then flex your feet, as if you're pumping a gas pedal. Repeat 15-20 times on each foot. This helps improve circulation and prevent stiffness in your ankles.

- **Wall Slides:** Stand facing a wall with your feet shoulder-width apart. Lean forward and place your hands on the wall at shoulder height. Slowly bend your knees, sliding your back down the wall until your thighs are parallel to the floor. Hold for a few seconds, then slowly slide back up. Repeat 10-15 times.

- **Desk Push-ups:** Stand facing your desk with your hands shoulder-width apart on the edge.

Lean forward and lower your chest towards the desk, bending your elbows. Push back up to the starting position. Repeat 10-15 times. This is a modified push-up that can help strengthen your arms, chest, and core.

The key is to move regularly throughout the day. Set a timer to remind yourself to get up and move every 30-60 minutes. Even a few minutes of movement can make a big difference in your knee health and overall well-being.

Additional Tips for Knee Health at Work

Beyond ergonomics and movement breaks, there are additional strategies you can incorporate into your workday to optimize your knee health and minimize discomfort:

- **Staying Hydrated:** Water is essential for joint lubrication and overall health. Aim to drink plenty of water throughout the day, especially if you're physically active or working in a warm environment. Dehydration can lead to thicker synovial fluid, which can reduce joint lubrication and increase friction, potentially contributing to pain and stiffness.

- **Wearing Comfortable Shoes:** Your choice of footwear can significantly impact your knee health. Opt for comfortable shoes that provide adequate support and cushioning. Avoid high heels or shoes with minimal support, as they can alter your posture and put extra strain on your knees. If you have specific foot conditions or biomechanical issues, consider consulting a podiatrist for recommendations on specialized footwear or custom orthotics.

- **Managing Stress:** Stress isn't just a mental burden; it can manifest physically, including in your joints. When you're stressed, your body releases hormones like cortisol, which can trigger inflammation and exacerbate pain. Find healthy ways to manage stress, such as mindfulness meditation, deep breathing exercises, or spending time in nature. By reducing stress, you're not only improving your mental well-being but also supporting your knee health.

- **Listening to Your Body:** Your body is constantly sending you signals, and it's important to pay attention to them. If you experience pain, stiffness, or fatigue in your knees, don't ignore it. Take a break, adjust your posture, or modify your activity. Pushing through pain can worsen existing problems and lead to further injury. Remember, your body knows best, so listen to its cues and prioritize rest and recovery when needed.

Creating a workspace that prioritizes your well-being is an investment in your long-term knee health. Even seemingly small adjustments to your daily routine and work environment can significantly reduce strain and prevent pain. Take the time to assess your workspace and make the necessary changes to create an environment that supports your knees and overall health. Your body will reap the rewards for years to come.

ACTION STEP: Put mineral salt in your drinking water to stay properly hydrated.

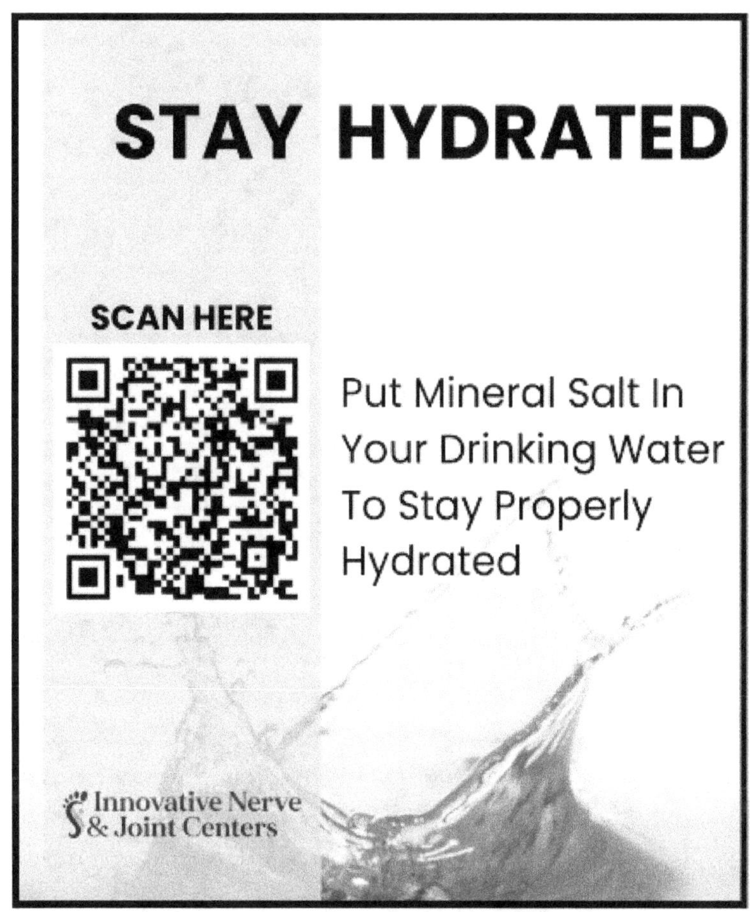

Unlock Your Path To Knee Pain Relief Now: Call (833) 359-6099 To Speak With An Expert Today!

5

PREVENTING KNEE INJURIES IN
SPORTS AND EXERCISE

David, a seasoned marathon runner, limped into my office, his face a mask of disappointment. "I was training for my tenth marathon," he explained, his voice tinged with frustration, "but this nagging knee pain just won't go away. I'm worried I'll have to give up running altogether." David's passion for running was evident, and the thought of abandoning it was clearly devastating. He'd tried rest, ice, and over-the-counter pain relievers, but the pain persisted, threatening to sideline him indefinitely.

David's assessment revealed a common issue among runners: IT band syndrome, coupled with weakness in his glutes and core. We implemented the FREEDOM Protocol, focusing on targeted exercises to strengthen these supporting muscles and improve his running mechanics. We also incorporated soft tissue work to release tension in his IT band and improve flexibility.

Weeks later, David bounded into my office, a wide grin replacing his previous grimace. "I'm back on track, Dr. Fisher!" he announced, practically vibrating with energy. "The pain is gone, and I'm running faster and stronger than before. I even signed up for another marathon!" Of course, David knows that not everyone experiences such significant improvements, and individual results can vary. His story, however, offers a beacon of hope, demonstrating that with the right approach, even persistent knee pain can be overcome.

This testimonial is not intended to represent typical results.

David's case highlights a critical point: knee injuries are a common hurdle for athletes and active individuals. However, understanding these injuries and taking proactive steps toward prevention and recovery can be the key to reclaiming your active lifestyle.

Understanding Knee Injuries in Athletes and Active Individuals

Knee injuries are a common setback for athletes and active individuals alike. They can sideline you from your favorite activities, cause significant pain, and even lead to long-term complications if not properly addressed. Understanding the common types of knee injuries is the first step in prevention and recovery. Let's take a closer look at some of the most frequent culprits:

- **Ligament Sprains and Tears:** Your knee joint is stabilized by four major ligaments: the anterior cruciate ligament (ACL), medial collateral ligament (MCL), posterior cruciate ligament (PCL), and lateral collateral ligament (LCL). These tough bands of tissue can be sprained (overstretched) or torn due to sudden twists, pivots, or impacts. ACL tears are particularly notorious among athletes, often requiring surgery and extensive rehabilitation.
- **Meniscus Tears:** The menisci are C-shaped pieces of cartilage that act as shock absorbers in your knee joint. They can tear due to forceful twisting or degeneration over time. Meniscus tears often cause pain, swelling, and a catching or locking sensation in the knee.
- **Tendonitis:** Tendons are the strong cords that connect muscles to bones. Overuse or repetitive strain can lead to inflammation and irritation of the tendons around your knee, such as patellar tendonitis (jumper's knee) or quadriceps tendonitis. Tendonitis typically

causes pain and tenderness around the affected tendon, especially during or after activity.

- **Runner's Knee (Patellofemoral Pain Syndrome):** This common overuse injury affects the cartilage under your kneecap (patella). It often causes pain around or behind the kneecap, especially when going up or down stairs, squatting, or kneeling.
- **Iliotibial (IT) Band Syndrome:** The IT band is a thick band of tissue that runs along the outside of your thigh, from your hip to your knee. Overuse or tightness in the IT band can cause friction and inflammation, leading to pain on the outer side of the knee, especially during activities like running or cycling.

Understanding these common knee injuries is crucial for prevention and early intervention. By recognizing the symptoms and seeking appropriate treatment, you can minimize the impact of these injuries and get back to doing what you love.

While some factors are beyond your control, many can be mitigated with awareness and proactive measures. Let's delve into the key risk factors that can increase your vulnerability to knee injuries:

- **Previous Knee Injuries:** If you've injured your knee in the past, you're more susceptible to future problems. Scar tissue, weakened ligaments, or altered movement patterns can create vulnerabilities that need to be addressed through targeted rehabilitation and strengthening exercises.

- **Muscle Imbalances and Weaknesses:** Imbalances in the strength and flexibility of the muscles surrounding your knee joint can disrupt its normal mechanics and increase the risk of injury. For example, weak hip muscles can lead to poor knee alignment and increased stress on the joint.

- **Poor Flexibility:** Tight muscles and limited range of motion in your hips, knees, and ankles can hinder your movement efficiency and put extra strain on your knee joint. Regular stretching and mobility exercises are essential for maintaining optimal flexibility.

- **Improper Training Techniques:** Using incorrect form during exercises or sports activities can place excessive stress on your knees. It's crucial to learn proper techniques and seek guidance from qualified professionals to ensure you're moving safely and efficiently.

- **Overuse and Overtraining:** Pushing your body too hard without adequate rest and recovery can lead to overuse injuries. Gradually increasing the intensity and duration of your activities and incorporating rest days into your training schedule are essential for preventing knee problems.

- **Sudden Increases in Activity Intensity or Duration:** A sudden spike in your training volume or intensity can shock your body and increase the risk of injury. Gradually progressing your workouts and allowing your body time to adapt is key.

- **Inadequate Warm-up or Cool-down:** Skipping a proper warm-up or cool-down can leave your muscles and joints unprepared for activity or hinder recovery. A good warm-up should include dynamic stretches and light cardio, while a cool-down should involve static stretches and relaxation techniques.

- **Playing on Hard or Uneven Surfaces:** Hard surfaces like concrete or uneven terrain can increase the impact on your knees. Whenever possible, choose softer surfaces like tracks or trails for running and sports activities.

- **Wearing Improper Footwear:** Shoes that lack support, cushioning, or proper fit can contribute to knee pain and injuries. Invest in quality footwear that matches your foot type and the demands of your chosen activities.

Prevention is always better than cure, and a little knowledge and effort can go a long way in safeguarding your knee health.

The Importance of a Comprehensive Warm-up

A well-structured warm-up is crucial for priming your body for the demands of exercise and significantly reducing the risk of knee injuries. Think of it as gradually waking up your muscles and joints, preparing them for the challenges ahead.

Preparing Your Body for Activity

The primary goal of a warm-up is to gradually increase your heart rate, blood flow, and muscle temperature. This prepares your cardiovascular system for the increased demands of exercise and enhances the elasticity of your muscles and connective tissues. A proper warm-up can improve your range of motion, making your movements smoother and more efficient, and reducing the likelihood of strains or tears.

Dynamic Stretches for Knee Injury Prevention

Dynamic stretches involve controlled movements that take your joints through their full range of motion. Unlike static stretches (holding a position), dynamic stretches mimic the movements you'll be performing during your workout, making them an ideal way to prepare your knees for activity. Here are some effective dynamic stretches for knee injury prevention:

- **Leg Swings:** Stand tall and gently swing one leg forward and backward, gradually increasing the range of motion. Repeat with the other leg. Then, swing each leg side to side, keeping your core engaged.
- **High Knees:** While jogging in place, bring your knees up towards your chest, alternating legs. This warms up your hip flexors and quadriceps.
- **Butt Kicks:** While jogging in place, kick your heels up towards your glutes, alternating legs. This activates your hamstrings and glutes.
- **Walking Lunges:** Step forward with one leg and lower your body until both knees are bent at a 90-degree angle. Push back up to the starting position and repeat with the other leg. This engages your quads, hamstrings, and glutes while improving hip mobility.

- **Arm Circles:** Extend your arms out to the sides and make small circles, gradually increasing the size of the circles. Reverse the direction. This warms up your shoulders and upper body, promoting overall mobility.

Foam Rolling and Self-Myofascial Release

Foam rolling is a form of self-myofascial release (SMR) that involves using a foam roller to massage your muscles and connective tissues. This technique can help release muscle tightness, improve flexibility, and reduce the risk of injury. For knee health, focus on rolling your quadriceps, hamstrings, calves, and IT band. Apply gentle pressure and roll slowly over each muscle group, pausing on any areas that feel particularly tight or tender.

By incorporating a comprehensive warm-up routine into your exercise regimen, you're not only enhancing your performance but also taking a proactive step towards protecting your knees from injury. Remember, a few minutes of preparation can save you weeks or even months of pain and rehabilitation.

Strength Training for Knee Stability

Building a strong foundation of muscles around your knee joint is like constructing a fortress to protect it from harm. These muscles act as dynamic stabilizers, absorbing shock, controlling movement, and reducing the stress placed on the ligaments and cartilage within the knee. Let's explore how to fortify this fortress and safeguard your knees:

Building a Strong Foundation

The key players in knee stability are your quadriceps (front of the thigh), hamstrings (back of the thigh), glutes (buttocks), and calves. Strengthening these muscle groups creates a supportive network that helps your knee joint function optimally and withstand the demands of daily activities and exercise.

Key Exercises for Knee Injury Prevention

Here are some fundamental exercises that target the muscles essential for knee stability:

- **Squats:** This compound movement engages multiple muscle groups, including your quads, hamstrings, and glutes. It mimics the natural movement of sitting and standing, making it a functional exercise for everyday life.

- **Lunges:** Lunges challenge your balance and coordination while strengthening your quads, hamstrings, and glutes. They also help improve hip mobility, which is crucial for proper knee alignment.
- **Step-ups:** This exercise targets your quads and glutes while also working on single-leg stability. It's a great way to improve balance and coordination, which are essential for preventing falls and knee injuries.
- **Hamstring Curls:** Hamstring curls isolate the muscles on the back of your thigh, which are important for knee stability and preventing ACL injuries. You can perform this exercise using a machine, resistance band, or bodyweight.
- **Calf Raises:** Strong calf muscles contribute to ankle stability, which in turn affects knee alignment and function. Calf raises are a simple yet effective way to strengthen these muscles.

Proper Form and Technique

While these exercises are beneficial, using improper form can negate their positive effects and even put your knees at risk. It's crucial to prioritize proper technique over the amount of weight lifted or the number of repetitions performed. If you're unsure about your form, consult with a qualified professional like a physical therapist or certified trainer. They can guide you through the correct movements and ensure you're getting the most out of your workouts while minimizing the risk of injury.

Progressive Overload

As your muscles get stronger, it's important to gradually increase the challenge to continue seeing progress. This principle, known as progressive overload, involves gradually increasing the intensity, duration, or frequency of your workouts over time. This can be achieved by adding weight, increasing repetitions, or trying more challenging variations of the exercises. Progressive overload ensures that your muscles continue to adapt and grow stronger, providing even greater support and protection for your knees.

Flexibility and Mobility for Knee Health

Flexibility and mobility are essential components of knee health, often overlooked in favor of strength training. Maintaining a full range of motion in your hips, knees, and ankles is crucial for preventing muscle tightness, joint stiffness, and ultimately, knee injuries. Let's explore how flexibility and mobility can benefit your knees and how to incorporate them into your routine:

The Importance of Maintaining Full Range of Motion

Think of your joints like hinges on a door. If the hinges are rusty and stiff, the door won't open and close smoothly. Similarly, if your joints lack flexibility, your movements become restricted and inefficient. This can lead to compensatory patterns, where other muscles and joints have to work harder to make up for the lack of mobility, increasing the risk of strain and injury.

Maintaining flexibility in the muscles and connective tissues around your knee joint allows for smooth, fluid movement. This reduces stress on the joint itself and promotes better circulation, which is essential for delivering nutrients and removing waste products. Additionally, flexibility can improve your balance and coordination, further reducing the risk of falls and injuries.

Stretches for Knee Injury Prevention

Incorporating regular stretching into your routine can significantly improve your flexibility and protect your knees. Here are some key stretches to focus on:

- **Quadriceps Stretch:** Stand tall and hold onto a wall or chair for balance. Bend one knee and bring your heel towards your buttock. Gently pull your heel closer until you feel a stretch in the front of your thigh. Hold for 30 seconds and repeat on the other side.

- **Hamstring Stretch:** As mentioned in the previous chapter, sit on the floor with one leg extended and the other bent. Reach towards your toes on the extended leg, keeping your back straight. You should feel a stretch in the back of your thigh. Hold for 30 seconds and repeat on the other side.
- **Calf Stretch:** Stand facing a wall with your hands on the wall at shoulder height. Step one foot back, keeping your heel on the ground and your knee straight. Lean forward until you feel a stretch in the back of your lower leg. Hold for 30 seconds and repeat on the other side.
- **Hip Flexor Stretch:** Kneel on one knee with the other foot flat on the floor in front of you. Gently push your hips forward until you feel a stretch in the front of your hip and thigh. Hold for 30 seconds and repeat on the other side.
- **IT Band Stretch:** Stand tall and cross one leg in front of the other. Lean towards the side of the crossed leg, reaching your opposite arm overhead. You should feel a stretch along the

outside of your hip and thigh. Hold for 30 seconds and repeat on the other side.

Yoga and Pilates for Flexibility and Balance

Yoga and Pilates are excellent mind-body practices that can enhance your flexibility, mobility, and balance. These disciplines emphasize controlled movements, core strength, and body awareness, all of which contribute to healthier knees. Consider incorporating yoga or Pilates classes into your routine to complement your stretching and strengthening exercises.

Remember, consistency is key when it comes to flexibility and mobility. Aim to stretch regularly, ideally after your workouts when your muscles are warm and pliable. Listen to your body and never push yourself into pain. If you have any concerns or limitations, consult with a physical therapist or qualified instructor for guidance and modifications.

Listening to Your Body and Avoiding Overtraining

In the pursuit of stronger, healthier knees, it's easy to get caught up in the excitement of progress and push your body beyond its limits. However, listening to your body and respecting its need for rest and recovery is just as crucial as the workouts themselves. Ignoring these signals can lead to overtraining, setbacks, and even injuries. Let's explore how to strike the right balance and ensure your knee health journey is sustainable and enjoyable:

Recognizing the Signs of Fatigue and Overexertion

Your body has a remarkable way of communicating its needs, but it's up to you to pay attention. Here are some common signs that you might be overdoing it:

- **Pain**: This is your body's most obvious alarm bell. Pain during or after exercise, especially if it's sharp or persistent, is a clear sign that something is wrong. Don't try to "push through" pain – it's a signal to back off and reassess.
- **Swelling**: Increased swelling in your knee joint can indicate inflammation and potential damage. If you notice persistent swelling, it's important to rest and allow your body to heal.
- **Stiffness**: Feeling unusually stiff or restricted in your knee joint can be a sign of overuse. Take a break from strenuous activity and focus on gentle movement and stretching.
- **Decreased Performance**: If you're struggling to maintain your usual pace or intensity during workouts, it could be a sign of fatigue. Listen to

your body and scale back your training if needed.

The Importance of Rest and Recovery

Rest and recovery are not signs of weakness; they're essential components of any training program. When you exercise, you create microscopic tears in your muscle fibers. Rest allows your body to repair these tears, making your muscles stronger and more resilient. It also gives your joints a chance to recover from the stress of exercise.

Incorporating Rest Days into Your Training Schedule

Rest days don't mean lying on the couch all day (although that's okay occasionally!). Active recovery, such as gentle yoga, swimming, or walking, can promote blood flow and aid in the healing process. Aim to incorporate at least one or two rest days into your weekly schedule, depending on the intensity and frequency of your workouts.

Modifying Your Activity When Needed

If you're feeling fatigued or experiencing pain, don't hesitate to modify your activity. This might mean reducing the intensity or duration of your workout, switching to a lower-impact activity, or taking a complete rest day. Remember, it's better to take a step back and allow your body to recover than to risk further injury.

Seeking Professional Guidance

If you're unsure how to balance activity and rest, or if you're experiencing persistent pain or other concerns, consult with a physical therapist or qualified trainer. We can assess your individual needs, create a personalized training plan, and offer guidance on how to listen to your body and avoid overtraining.

Additional Tips for Knee Injury Prevention

In addition to the foundational elements of warm-up, strength training, and flexibility, there are several additional strategies you can implement to further safeguard your knees and minimize the risk of injury:

- **Wearing Proper Footwear:** Your shoes are your first line of defense against impact and stress. Choose footwear that provides adequate support, cushioning, and stability for your specific activity. Replace worn-out shoes regularly, as their shock-absorbing capabilities diminish over time. If you have specific foot conditions or biomechanical issues, consider consulting a podiatrist for recommendations on specialized footwear or custom orthotics.

- **Maintaining a Healthy Weight:** Excess weight places a significant burden on your knees. Each extra pound you carry translates to several pounds of additional force on your joints with every step. Maintaining a healthy weight through a balanced diet and regular exercise can significantly reduce stress on your knees and lower your risk of injury.

- **Using Proper Technique in Sports and Activities:** Whether you're playing a sport, lifting weights, or simply going for a walk, using proper technique is crucial for protecting your knees. Avoid sudden twisting or pivoting motions, land softly when jumping, and focus on maintaining good form during exercises. If you're unsure about proper technique, seek guidance from a qualified professional.

- **Gradually Increasing Activity Levels:** Avoid the temptation to jump into intense activity without proper preparation. Gradually increase the intensity, duration, and frequency of your workouts over time. This allows your body to adapt and build strength and resilience, minimizing the risk of overuse injuries.

- **Cross-Training**: Incorporating a variety of activities into your routine can help prevent overuse injuries by distributing stress across different muscle groups and joints. For example, if you're a runner, consider adding swimming or cycling to your training plan to give your knees a break from the repetitive impact of running.

By implementing these additional strategies alongside a comprehensive warm-up, strength training, and flexibility routine, you can create a multi-layered approach to knee injury prevention. Remember, your knees are remarkable joints capable of supporting you through a lifetime of activity. By taking proactive steps to protect them, you can enjoy a future of pain-free movement and continue pursuing the activities you love.

ACTION STEP: Get the Little-Known Secrets to Reversing Knee Pain by scanning the code below.

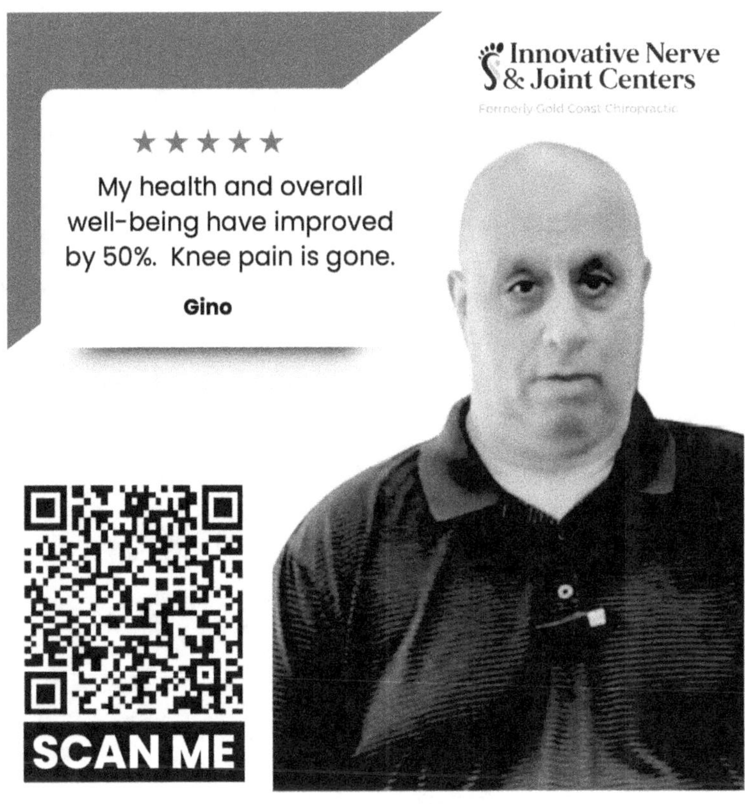

Unlock Your Path To Knee Pain Relief Now: Call (833) 359-6099 To Speak With An Expert Today!

6

———

KNEE PAIN IN SPECIAL POPULATIONS

Maria, a vibrant 70-year-old, entered my office with a hesitant gait, her hand resting on her grandson's arm. "My knees are just worn out," she said with a sigh, "It's just part of getting older, isn't it?" Maria had gradually limited her activities, resigning herself to a life with less movement and more pain. She missed her weekly Zumba classes and the simple joy of playing with her grandchildren without wincing. She believed, like many older adults, that knee pain was an inevitable consequence of aging, something she simply had to accept.

Maria's story touched my heart. I knew that while age-related changes can contribute to knee pain, it doesn't have to dictate the quality of your life. We discussed the FREEDOM Protocol, emphasizing our personalized approach. Her assessment revealed osteoarthritis in both knees, coupled with decreased muscle strength and flexibility. We developed a tailored plan that combined gentle, low-impact exercises with targeted strength training and mobility work. We also addressed her nutritional needs, focusing on anti-inflammatory foods to support her joint health.

Months later, Maria returned, her transformation astounding. She walked in unassisted, a radiant smile illuminating her face. "I feel like a new woman!" she exclaimed. "I'm back to Zumba, and I can chase after my grandkids without a second thought. I never imagined I could feel this good again." I always remind patients that while Maria's experience is inspiring, individual outcomes can differ.

This is one individual's experience and does not guarantee similar results.

Maria's story is a powerful reminder that while knee pain is a common complaint, the experience is far from universal.

Understanding Unique Needs

Knee pain is a common complaint, but it's important to recognize that it's not a one-size-fits-all condition. Different populations experience knee pain in unique ways, influenced by factors like age, underlying health conditions, and lifestyle. Understanding these unique needs is crucial for developing effective and personalized treatment plans.

The Impact of Aging on Knee Health

As we age, our bodies undergo natural changes that can affect our knee health. These changes can increase our susceptibility to knee pain and require adjustments to our approach to exercise, nutrition, and pain management.

- **Increased Prevalence of Osteoarthritis and Other Degenerative Conditions:** Osteoarthritis, a wear-and-tear condition affecting the cartilage in our joints, becomes more common with age. Other degenerative conditions like meniscus tears and tendonitis can also contribute to knee pain in older adults.
- **Decreased Muscle Mass and Strength:** Age-related muscle loss, known as sarcopenia, can weaken the muscles that support our knees, making them more vulnerable to injury and pain.
- **Reduced Flexibility and Mobility:** Our joints naturally become stiffer as we age, leading to

decreased range of motion and increased risk of injury.

- **Other Age-Related Health Conditions:** Conditions like diabetes, obesity, and cardiovascular disease can exacerbate knee pain and complicate treatment.

It's important to note that these changes don't mean that knee pain is an inevitable part of aging. With proactive measures and appropriate care, older adults can maintain healthy knees and enjoy an active lifestyle. The key is to tailor your approach to your individual needs and limitations, focusing on low-impact activities, strength training, and flexibility exercises that are safe and effective for your age and fitness level.

Pregnancy and Knee Pain

Pregnancy is a time of remarkable transformation, but it can also bring about unexpected challenges, including knee pain. Several factors contribute to this discomfort, and understanding them is key to finding relief and maintaining an active, healthy pregnancy.

- **Hormonal Changes and Their Effects on Joints and Ligaments:** During pregnancy, your body releases hormones like relaxin, which helps prepare your pelvis for childbirth by loosening ligaments and joints. While this is essential for delivery, it can also lead to increased laxity (looseness) in other joints, including your knees. This can make your knees feel less stable and more prone to pain, especially during weight-bearing activities.

- **Weight Gain and Its Impact on Knee Stress:** As your baby grows, so does your body weight. This additional weight puts extra stress on your knees, particularly the cartilage that cushions the joint. The increased load can exacerbate existing knee problems or trigger new ones.

- **Postural Changes and Their Influence on Knee Alignment:** As your belly expands, your center of gravity shifts, often leading to changes in your posture. You might find yourself leaning back slightly to compensate for the extra weight in front. This can alter the alignment of your knees, putting uneven pressure on the joint and potentially leading to pain.

Knee pain during pregnancy is not uncommon, and it doesn't mean you have to give up on physical activity. In fact, staying active can be beneficial for both you and your baby. However, it's crucial to listen to your body, modify activities as needed, and seek guidance from your healthcare provider or a physical therapist specializing in prenatal care. We can help you develop a safe and effective exercise plan that supports your changing body and minimizes knee discomfort.

Medical Conditions and Knee Pain

Beyond age and pregnancy, various medical conditions can significantly contribute to knee pain, often requiring specialized care and tailored treatment approaches. Let's delve into some of these conditions:

- **Autoimmune Diseases (Rheumatoid Arthritis, Lupus):** These conditions involve the immune system mistakenly attacking the body's own tissues, including the joints. Rheumatoid arthritis, in particular, commonly affects the knees, causing inflammation, pain, stiffness, and potential joint damage. Lupus, while less likely to directly target the knees, can still cause joint pain and inflammation as part of its broader systemic effects.
- **Diabetes:** Individuals with diabetes are at increased risk of developing osteoarthritis, nerve damage (neuropathy), and poor circulation, all of which can contribute to knee

pain. High blood sugar levels can also accelerate cartilage degeneration and impair the body's ability to repair damaged tissues.

- **Obesity:** Excess weight places a significant burden on the knees, increasing the risk of osteoarthritis and other joint problems. The added stress on the cartilage can lead to faster wear and tear, pain, and inflammation.
- **Other Chronic Conditions:** Various other chronic conditions can contribute to knee pain, including gout (a type of arthritis caused by uric acid buildup), psoriasis (a skin condition that can also affect joints), and certain infections.

It's important to note that these conditions often require a multidisciplinary approach to manage knee pain effectively. This may involve collaboration between your primary care physician, rheumatologist, endocrinologist, or other specialists, along with physical therapists and pain management experts. The goal is to address both the underlying medical condition and the resulting knee pain through a combination of medication, lifestyle modifications, physical therapy, and other appropriate interventions.

Tailored Exercise Recommendations

Older Adults

For older adults experiencing knee pain, the key is to find a balance between staying active and protecting your joints. Low-impact activities, strength training, and flexibility exercises can all play a role in maintaining knee health and improving your quality of life.

Low-Impact Activities:

These activities are gentle on your joints while still providing cardiovascular benefits and helping to maintain a healthy weight. Some excellent options include:

- **Walking:** Start with shorter walks and gradually increase the distance and duration as your knees get stronger. Consider using walking poles for added stability and support.
- **Swimming:** The buoyancy of water reduces stress on your joints, making swimming an ideal exercise for people with knee pain. It provides a full-body workout without the impact of land-based activities.
- **Water Aerobics:** This fun and social activity combines the benefits of swimming with

targeted exercises to improve strength, flexibility, and cardiovascular health.

- **Cycling:** Whether outdoors or on a stationary bike, cycling is a low-impact way to get your heart rate up and strengthen your leg muscles.

Strength Training:

Building strength in the muscles surrounding your knees can improve stability, reduce pain, and prevent further injury. Focus on exercises that target your quadriceps, hamstrings, and glutes, such as:

- **Chair Squats:** Sit in a chair with your feet shoulder-width apart. Slowly stand up, using your leg muscles to lift your body. Slowly lower yourself back down to the chair. Repeat 10-15 times.
- **Wall Sits:** Stand with your back against a wall, feet shoulder-width apart. Slide down the wall until your thighs are parallel to the floor, as if you're sitting in an invisible chair. Hold for 30-60 seconds, then slowly slide back up.
- **Leg Presses:** This machine-based exercise allows you to strengthen your leg muscles without putting excessive stress on your knees. Start with a light weight and gradually increase the resistance as you get stronger.

Flexibility Exercises:

Gentle stretches can help maintain your range of motion, reduce stiffness, and prevent injuries. Focus on stretches that target your hamstrings, quadriceps, calves, and hips. Hold each stretch for 30 seconds and repeat 2-3 times.

Remember, it's always best to consult with your doctor or a physical therapist before starting any new exercise program. We can help you tailor a plan to your specific needs and abilities, ensuring that you're exercising safely and effectively.

Pregnant Women

Staying active during pregnancy offers numerous benefits for both mother and baby, including improved mood, reduced risk of gestational diabetes, and better postpartum recovery. However, it's crucial to exercise safely and adapt your routine to accommodate the changes your body is undergoing.

Prenatal Exercise Guidelines:

Before starting or continuing any exercise program during pregnancy, it's essential to consult with your healthcare provider. They can assess your individual health and risk factors and provide personalized recommendations for safe and appropriate activities.

Modified Exercises:

As your pregnancy progresses, you may need to modify your exercises to accommodate changes in your body, such as:

- **Reduced Intensity:** Listen to your body and avoid pushing yourself too hard. Lower the intensity of your workouts if you feel fatigued or experience any discomfort.
- **Modified Positions:** Avoid exercises that involve lying flat on your back, especially during the second and third trimesters. This position can put pressure on a major blood vessel and restrict blood flow to the baby. Opt for exercises that can be done in a seated, standing, or side-lying position.
- **Proper Form:** Pay close attention to your form and avoid any movements that strain your joints or ligaments. Use lighter weights or resistance bands if needed.

Avoiding High-Impact Activities:

High-impact activities like running, jumping, and contact sports can put excessive stress on your joints and increase the risk of injury. Opt for low-impact alternatives like:

- **Swimming:** The buoyancy of water supports your body weight, reducing stress on your joints. Swimming is a great way to get a full-body workout without the impact of land-based activities.
- **Prenatal Yoga:** This gentle form of yoga is specifically designed for pregnant women, focusing on stretches and poses that are safe and beneficial for both mother and baby.
- **Walking:** Walking is a low-impact exercise that can be easily adapted to your fitness level and stage of pregnancy.

Every pregnancy is different, and what works for one woman may not work for another. Listen to your body, prioritize your comfort and safety, and don't hesitate to seek guidance from your healthcare provider or a qualified prenatal exercise specialist.

Individuals with Medical Conditions

If you have a medical condition that affects your knees, exercise can still be a valuable tool for managing pain and improving function. However, it's crucial to work closely with your healthcare providers to develop a safe and effective exercise plan that takes your specific needs into account.

Working with Healthcare Providers:

Collaboration is key when it comes to exercise and medical conditions. Your doctor and physical therapist can assess your individual situation, considering factors like:

- **Type and Severity of Your Condition:** Different medical conditions require different approaches to exercise. For example, someone with rheumatoid arthritis might need to focus on low-impact activities and gentle range-of-motion exercises, while someone with diabetes might need to monitor their blood sugar levels closely during exercise.
- **Medications and Treatments:** Certain medications can affect your exercise tolerance or increase your risk of injury. Your healthcare providers can help you understand these potential interactions and adjust your exercise plan accordingly.
- **Current Fitness Level:** Your starting point will influence the type and intensity of exercises that are appropriate for you. Your physical therapist can help you gradually progress your workouts as your strength and endurance improve.

Modifying Exercises Based on Individual Needs:

Exercise modifications are often necessary for individuals with medical conditions. These modifications can involve:

- **Adjusting Intensity:** Lowering the intensity of exercises to avoid overexertion and minimize stress on your joints. This might involve using lighter weights, reducing the number of repetitions, or opting for lower-impact activities.
- **Duration:** Shortening the duration of your workouts or breaking them up into smaller, more frequent sessions. This can help prevent fatigue and reduce the risk of injury.
- **Type of Activity:** Choosing activities that are appropriate for your condition and fitness level. For example, if you have balance issues, you might avoid activities that require a lot of coordination.

Prioritizing Safety and Comfort:

Above all, it's essential to listen to your body and prioritize your safety and comfort. If an exercise causes pain or discomfort, stop immediately and consult with your healthcare provider. Don't push yourself beyond your limits, and remember that even gentle movement can be beneficial.

Nutritional Considerations for Special Populations

Older Adults

As we age, our nutritional needs evolve, and maintaining optimal knee health becomes even more crucial. A well-balanced, nutrient-dense diet can provide the building blocks for strong bones, healthy cartilage, and resilient joints. Let's explore the key nutritional considerations for older adults with knee pain:

- **Nutrient-Dense Diet:** Prioritize whole foods that are packed with essential vitamins, minerals, and antioxidants. These nutrients play a vital role in reducing inflammation, protecting cartilage, and supporting overall joint health. Fill your plate with colorful fruits and vegetables, whole grains, lean protein sources, and healthy fats.
- **Adequate Protein Intake:** Protein is essential for maintaining muscle mass and strength, which are crucial for supporting your knees and preventing injuries. Aim to include protein-rich foods like lean meats, fish, poultry,

beans, lentils, nuts, and seeds in your daily meals. If you struggle to meet your protein needs through diet alone, consider discussing protein supplements with your doctor or a registered dietitian.

- **Hydration:** Staying hydrated is often overlooked but incredibly important for joint health. Water helps lubricate your joints, transport nutrients, and flush out waste products. Aim to drink plenty of water throughout the day, especially if you're physically active or live in a warm climate. You can also get fluids from other sources like herbal teas, soups, and fruits and vegetables with high water content.

By focusing on these nutritional pillars, you're not only nourishing your body but also actively supporting your knee health. A well-balanced diet can reduce inflammation, protect cartilage, and strengthen the muscles that support your joints, leading to less pain, improved function, and a better quality of life.

Pregnant Women

Proper nutrition during pregnancy is vital for the health of both the mother and the developing baby. It also plays a crucial role in managing knee pain and supporting joint health during this transformative time.

Prenatal Nutrition Guidelines:

Following established prenatal nutrition guidelines is essential for ensuring you and your baby receive the necessary nutrients for optimal health. These guidelines typically include recommendations for:

- **Calorie Intake:** You'll need additional calories during pregnancy to support your baby's growth and development. However, it's important to avoid excessive weight gain, as this can put extra stress on your knees. Consult with your healthcare provider or a registered dietitian to determine your individual calorie needs.
- **Macronutrients:** Focus on a balanced intake of carbohydrates, protein, and healthy fats. Carbohydrates provide energy, protein supports tissue growth and repair, and healthy fats are essential for hormone production and brain development.
- **Micronutrients:** Certain vitamins and minerals are particularly important during pregnancy, such as folic acid, iron, calcium, and vitamin D. These nutrients play crucial roles in

fetal development, bone health, and overall well-being. Your healthcare provider may recommend prenatal vitamins to ensure you're getting adequate amounts of these essential nutrients.

Avoiding Inflammatory Foods:

Certain foods can trigger or worsen inflammation in the body, which can exacerbate knee pain. During pregnancy, it's especially important to limit or avoid:

- **Processed Foods:** These foods are often high in sugar, unhealthy fats, and artificial ingredients, which can contribute to inflammation.
- **Sugary Drinks:** Sugary sodas, juices, and energy drinks can lead to weight gain and inflammation. Opt for water, herbal teas, or unsweetened beverages instead.
- **Unhealthy Fats:** Limit your intake of saturated and trans fats, which are found in fried foods, processed snacks, and baked goods. Choose healthier fats like those found in avocados, nuts, seeds, and olive oil.

Staying Hydrated:

Staying hydrated is crucial during pregnancy, as your body's fluid needs increase to support the growing baby and amniotic fluid. Aim to drink plenty of water throughout the day, and listen to your body's thirst cues. Dehydration can lead to fatigue, headaches, and constipation, and it can also worsen joint pain.

Individuals with Medical Conditions

When managing knee pain alongside a medical condition, nutrition plays a crucial role in supporting overall health and minimizing inflammation, a common contributor to joint discomfort. However, dietary needs can vary significantly depending on the specific condition.

Dietary Modifications Based on Specific Conditions:

- **Rheumatoid Arthritis (RA):** Focus on anti-inflammatory foods like fatty fish, fruits, vegetables, and whole grains. Some individuals with RA find that eliminating nightshade vegetables (tomatoes, potatoes, peppers, eggplant) and gluten can help reduce inflammation and pain.
- **Lupus:** A balanced diet rich in fruits, vegetables, and whole grains is essential. Some

individuals with lupus may benefit from limiting saturated and trans fats, as well as refined sugars, which can trigger inflammation.

- **Diabetes:** Managing blood sugar levels is crucial for individuals with diabetes. A diet low in refined carbohydrates and added sugars, with a focus on fiber-rich foods like vegetables, fruits, and whole grains, can help regulate blood sugar and reduce inflammation.

- **Obesity:** A calorie-controlled diet that emphasizes nutrient-dense foods like fruits, vegetables, lean protein, and whole grains can help with weight management, which is essential for reducing stress on the knees.

Working with a Registered Dietitian:

Navigating dietary modifications for specific medical conditions can be complex. A registered dietitian can provide personalized guidance based on your individual needs, preferences, and health goals. They can help you create a meal plan that supports your overall health, manages your medical condition, and minimizes knee pain.

A registered dietitian can also help you identify potential food sensitivities or intolerances that may be contributing to your knee pain. They can guide you through elimination diets or other strategies to pinpoint trigger foods and develop a sustainable eating plan that promotes optimal health and well-being.

Pain Management Strategies

Effective pain management is crucial for individuals with knee pain, but the approach needs to be tailored to the specific needs and circumstances of each person. Let's explore pain management strategies for different populations:

Older Adults

- **Non-Pharmacological Approaches:** For older adults, prioritizing non-invasive pain management techniques is often the safest and most effective approach. These can include:
  - **Physical Therapy:** A physical therapist can design a personalized exercise program to strengthen muscles, improve flexibility, and reduce pain.
  - **Exercise:** Low-impact activities like walking, swimming, and tai chi can help manage pain and improve joint function.
  - **Heat/Cold Therapy:** Applying heat or cold

packs to the affected knee can help reduce inflammation and alleviate pain.

- **Other Non-Invasive Techniques:** Massage therapy, acupuncture, and transcutaneous electrical nerve stimulation (TENS) are other options that can be explored.

- **Medication Management:** While medications can be helpful for managing pain, it's important to work closely with your healthcare provider to choose the safest and most effective options. They can help you weigh the benefits and risks of different medications, considering potential interactions with other medications you may be taking.

Pregnant Women

- **Safe Pain Relief Options:** Pregnant women should always consult with their healthcare provider before taking any medication or undergoing any treatment for knee pain. Safe options may include:
  - **Physical Therapy:** A physical therapist can provide guidance on safe exercises and stretches to alleviate pain and improve function.

- ○ **Massage:** Prenatal massage can help reduce muscle tension and improve circulation, potentially easing knee discomfort.
  - ○ **Approved Over-the-Counter Medications:** Some over-the-counter pain relievers, like acetaminophen (Tylenol), may be considered safe during pregnancy, but it's crucial to discuss this with your doctor.
- **Avoiding Certain Medications and Therapies:** Some medications and therapies are not recommended during pregnancy due to potential risks to the developing fetus. These may include nonsteroidal anti-inflammatory drugs (NSAIDs) like ibuprofen (Advil) and naproxen (Aleve), as well as certain types of physical therapy modalities.

Individuals with Medical Conditions

- **Multidisciplinary Pain Management:** For individuals with underlying medical conditions, a multidisciplinary approach to pain management is often necessary. This involves collaboration between various healthcare providers, such as your primary care physician, specialists (e.g., rheumatologist, endocrinologist), physical therapists, and pain management specialists. This team can develop a comprehensive plan that addresses both the knee pain and the underlying condition.

- **Exploring Alternative Therapies:** In addition to conventional treatments, individuals with medical conditions may benefit from exploring alternative therapies like acupuncture, chiropractic care, and massage therapy. These approaches can complement traditional treatments and offer additional pain relief and improved function.

A holistic approach to knee health encompasses more than just exercise and ergonomics. It's about nourishing your body, managing stress, and tuning into your body's signals. These additional strategies, when combined with a well-rounded approach to movement and workplace modifications, can significantly enhance your knee health and overall well-being. A proactive approach is key to a more comfortable and fulfilling work life.

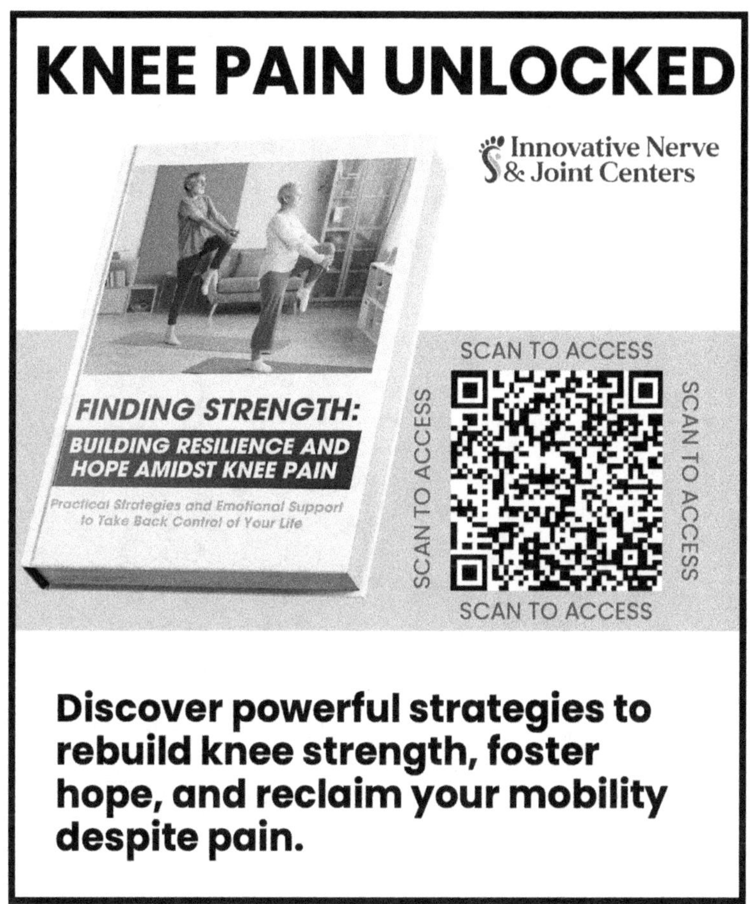

Unlock Your Path To Knee Pain Relief Now: Call (833) 359-6099 To Speak With An Expert Today!

7

INDIVIDUALIZED STABILITY EXERCISES

James, a high school basketball player, sat on my examination table, his leg braced and his dreams seemingly on hold. A recent ACL tear had sidelined him from the sport he loved, leaving him frustrated and uncertain about his future. "I just want to get back on the court," he said, his voice filled with a quiet determination that resonated with my own athletic past. He'd completed the initial round of physical therapy, but his knee still felt unstable, and he lacked the confidence to push himself. He worried that his injury would permanently impact his performance and potentially jeopardize his chances of playing college ball.

James's case highlighted the need for a more tailored approach. Standard rehabilitation protocols often follow a generic timeline, but every athlete's body heals and responds differently. With the FREEDOM Protocol, we delved deeper into James's specific needs. His assessment revealed lingering muscle imbalances and movement limitations. We designed a personalized exercise plan that focused on strengthening his core, improving his hip and ankle stability, and retraining his neuromuscular control. We gradually progressed the exercises, challenging him while respecting his body's limitations. Of course, I reminded James that everyone's journey to recovery is different, and his experience isn't a guarantee of similar outcomes for others.

Individual outcomes may differ.

Months later, James sent me a video of himself back on the court, executing a flawless jump shot. The sheer joy on his face was enough to make my day. His story underscores a fundamental principle of the FREEDOM Protocol:

Customization is Key

Personalized Exercise: The Key in FREEDOM

Think of your body as a complex and unique machine. What works for one person might not deliver the same results for another. This is especially true with knee health and stability. The FREEDOM program understands this, which is why personalized exercise plans lie at its core. Injury histories, movement patterns, flexibility levels, and even your current fitness all shape a training plan that's designed to work specifically for you.

Tailored Plans: Why They Win

One-size-fits-all stability exercise programs are out there, but they often fall short. Why? They may be suitable as a starting point, but they don't evolve with your progress. A generic program can't address your specific imbalances or weaknesses. With an individualized plan, you're not just following a routine – you're targeting the areas that will truly make a difference for your knees in the long term.

Let's dig deeper into why tailored plans hold an edge over cookie-cutter workouts for stability:

- **No Two Knees Are Alike (even your own):** Even with the same diagnosis, like osteoarthritis, two people's knees will be in different states. Inflammation levels, pain locations, and the surrounding muscles' strength all vary. A generic program can't consider these nuances. It might be too easy for some, risking boredom and lack of progress, or too difficult for others, increasing frustration and the potential for injury.

- **Addressing Imbalances:** Muscle imbalances are common, especially after an injury. For example, your quads might be strong, but your glutes might be underutilized. A one-size-fits-all program might have you doing lots of squats, further strengthening the already dominant quads instead of targeting the weaker areas for balanced stability.

- **Movement Patterns Matter:** How you move is just as important as what muscles you engage. Maybe you have a habit of letting your knees cave inwards during exercises. A generic program won't pick up on this, but a tailored plan can include exercises specifically designed to retrain your movement patterns for long-term knee health.

- **Adapting Over Time:** As you get stronger and more stable, your body needs new challenges to keep improving. A cookie-cutter program remains the same, leading to plateaus. Individualized plans introduce progressions - whether that's more difficult variations, increased weights, or new exercises altogether.

The Bottom Line: A generic program might give you a little improvement initially, but it won't unlock your full potential or bring the lasting benefits that a well-designed, individualized stability plan can. The personalized approach is a targeted investment in your knee health.

Build Your Stability Routine

Building your personalized stability plan doesn't need to be intimidating. Think of it as a three-step process to set your journey in motion:

1. **Self-Assessment Time:** Be honest with yourself about your current abilities. Try a simple test: Can you balance on one leg for 10 seconds? How does a basic squat feel? If certain movements are difficult or painful, take note. This isn't about judgment, but about creating a baseline to measure your progress against.

2. **Goals That Spark Motivation:** "I want to be more stable" is too vague. Picture what you want to be able to do: pain-free walks around your neighborhood, playing tag with your grandkids, or finally tackling that scenic hiking trail. The more specific your goal, the easier it is to tailor your exercise plan to achieve it.

3. **Seek Expert Guidance (Even If It's Just Once):**
   While you might ultimately do your exercises
   at home, an initial consultation with a physical
   therapist or experienced trainer is invaluable.
   We can help you understand where your weak
   areas truly lie, identify any movement patterns
   that might be harming your knees, and suggest
   exercises that are both safe and effective for
   your specific situation.

Remember, your stability exercise plan isn't set in stone.
As you progress within the FREEDOM program, your
plan will change and adapt alongside you.

Building a Foundation of Strength

Core Strength: Your Knee's Best Friend

When you think of knee pain, your core muscles
might not be the first thing that comes to mind. But
the truth is, a strong core is utterly essential for
supporting healthy, stable knees. Picture your core as
a sturdy pillar – it stabilizes your spine, pelvis, and
hips, all of which have a direct impact on how your
knees move and bear weight. Weak core muscles can
lead to all sorts of problems for your knees, from
improper movement patterns to increased strain on
the joints.

The Core Isn't Just About Abs

While we often imagine the "six-pack" muscles when talking about the core, it goes much deeper. It's a complex network of muscles including your deep abdominals (like the transverse abdominis), back muscles, hip flexors, glutes, and even your diaphragm. Think of these as the inner scaffolding for your whole body.

Stability, Not Just Strength

Your core isn't just about powering you through sit-ups. It's really about stability. When your core is strong, your spine, pelvis, and hips have a solid foundation. This has a direct impact on your legs, including your knees:

- **Alignment is Key:** Proper knee alignment depends on a stable core. If your core is weak, your pelvis might tilt, or your hips might rotate slightly, leading to your knees twisting inward or buckling awkwardly. Over time, this misalignment puts unnecessary stress on your knee joints.
- **Shock Absorption:** Your core plays a role in how well your body handles impact. Think about jumping – a strong core helps you land correctly, distributing the force instead of letting all the shock go straight to your knees.

It's a Chain Reaction

Weakness in one area often means other parts of your body have to compensate. Weak core muscles might lead to over-reliance on your quads, putting added strain on the knee joint. Or tight hip flexors caused by a weak core can pull on your pelvis, again throwing off your knee alignment.

The Bottom Line: If you're dealing with knee pain, don't ignore your core. Strengthening those deep stabilizing muscles can create a cascade of positive effects for your knees. You might be surprised at how much of a difference it makes!

Invest in Stability, Protect Your Knees

You may think that strengthening your core has nothing to do with your knees, but it's one of the most proactive things you can do for the long-term health of your knees. Think of a strong, stable core as a hidden superpower: subtly but strongly supporting every step you take.

Consider how your knees feel after standing all day. A good core helps your body manage that load better. The ability to share the loads correctly within the body ensures equal distribution of the large forces involved in walking, running, and even simple long-term standing. This could save the knees from tiny pieces generating wear and tear over a lifetime.

This brings me to the second important point. A strong core is needed for proper alignment throughout the body. With a well-aligned pelvis and spine, the knees track smoothly—without all the awful twists and torques that are so hard on cartilage and ligaments. This is crucial for protecting structures that make it possible for you to move without pain.

And the benefits aren't confined to your knees. A good core will additionally improve your posture, which translates into a lowering of the amount of stress placed on the rest of your body. It's also simpler to maintain superb balance, cutting your chances of falling. Every daily task becomes easier when you have to run errands or play tag with your grandkids.

The hours invested in making your core stronger now pay off exponentially when you're older. It's a simple way to ensure greater mobility, less pain, and the ability to remain active doing the things you love as the years go by.

Knee Pain Starter Kit: Build Your Core

Ready to give your knees the support they crave? These beginner-friendly exercises are a great place to start your core strengthening journey:

- **Planks:** Aim to hold a strong, straight line from head to heels. It sounds simple, but really focus on engaging those deep abdominal muscles. If a full plank is intense, start with a modified version on your knees, or holding for shorter periods of time. This can even be modified to do against a wall if getting up from the floor is a concern.

- **Bird Dogs:** Extend your opposite arm and leg out straight, keeping your core super tight to prevent your lower back from arching. This challenges your stability in multiple ways. Start with shorter holds if needed, and focus on controlled movements.

- **Glute Bridges:** Lie on your back, then lift your hips, squeezing your glutes at the top. This might look like a lower body exercise, but trust me, it fires up your core too!

- **Dead bug:** Lie on your back with knees bent and feet flat on the floor. Extend one arm overhead and the opposite leg out straight, keeping your core engaged. Slowly return to the starting position and repeat on the other side. This is great for coordination and those deep core muscles that support your spine.

- **Side Plank (Modified):** Start on your side, propped on your forearm with knees bent and stacked. Gently lift your hips so your body forms a side line, but keep your bottom knee on the floor for support. Hold, then switch sides. This targets those side abdominals (obliques) that are important for stability.

- **Wall sits:** Stand with your back against a wall, feet shoulder-width apart. Slide down until your thighs are parallel to the floor, as if sitting in an invisible chair. Hold, then slide back up. This is a quad burner, but it engages your core as it works to keep your spine pressed against the wall.

Important Notes:

- **Listen to Your Body:** If any exercise causes sharp pain in your knees, stop immediately. There might be a modification that works better for you, or you might need to consult a physical therapist before proceeding.
- **Focus on Form:** Proper technique is key to getting the benefits and avoiding injury. If you're unsure, watching a quick instructional video online or even doing a session with a trainer to check your form can be incredibly helpful.

- **Progression:** As you get stronger, try the full versions of these exercises (no more kneeling planks!). You can also increase the hold times, add repetitions, or even incorporate light weights for an extra challenge.
- **Resources:** There's a wealth of video tutorials on YouTube demonstrating these exercises, making it easy to learn the correct form.

Adapting to Change

Stability Training: Leveling Up

The beauty of the FREEDOM program is that it's designed to adjust along with your progress. The same goes for your stability exercises. As you get stronger and more confident, your plan needs to change to keep challenging you. Think of it as leveling up!

Progress = Customization

Remember when a basic plank felt like a major victory? That's the beauty of progression. As you get stronger, you can unlock new variations of your favorite stability exercises, bringing fresh challenges and even greater results. Let's look at some examples:

- **Plank:** You started on your knees, feeling that deep core burn. Then, you conquered the classic full plank. Now, the possibilities are exciting! Try alternating leg lifts to introduce a balance element, or a single arm lift for an even greater challenge. Once you're truly a plank pro, the side plank variation opens a whole new world of core strength.

- **Bird Dog:** Mastering that opposite arm-and-leg extension is a milestone in itself. To take it further, try adding light wrist or ankle weights to increase the resistance. Holding the position for longer durations builds endurance. Want a real test? Close your eyes! Removing your visual reference forces your core to go into overdrive to maintain your balance.

- **Glute Bridge:** Once you've nailed the basic glute bridge, here's how to level up:
    - Single-Leg Bridge: Lift one leg straight upwards, keeping hips level. This requires even more glute and core control.
    - March Variation: At the top of your bridge, slowly lower one heel towards your butt, then return to the top position. Repeat on the other side.
    - Weighted Option: Hold a light dumbbell or a sturdy object (like a water bottle) across your hips for added resistance.

- **Squats:** This isn't purely a core exercise, but strong core stability is essential for proper form. Progress your basic squat by:
  - Narrowing Your Stance: A narrower stance increases the balance challenge, working those stabilizing muscles harder.
  - Tempo Change: Slow down your squat, focusing on control throughout the movement.
  - Adding Weight: Hold dumbbells or a kettlebell to increase the resistance and demand more from your core.
- **Adding Instability:** Many stability exercises can be made more challenging by introducing an unstable surface:
  - Balance Pad: Perfect for planks, bird dogs, even single-leg exercises.
  - BOSU Ball: Great for modifying squats, adding a balance element to push-ups, and much more.

Remember, progression is individual! If these variations feel too difficult, there are often ways to scale them back down. Always listen to your body and seek guidance from a physical therapist if you're unsure.

Adaptability: Your Knee Health Superpower

Your body is incredibly adaptable. While this helps you master new skills initially, it can also lead to plateaus if you don't change things up. The same goes for stability exercises. Repeating the exact routine with the same intensity will eventually stop yielding the same results. That's why it's crucial to keep your workouts fresh. Not only does this help fight boredom (which is key for staying motivated!), but it also exposes hidden weaknesses. As you get stronger, your body can find ways to compensate; switching up your exercises forces those underworked muscles to step up.

This consistent challenge is what builds long-term resilience and knee health. You're improving more than just strength – you're honing your balance, coordination, and the ability to react quickly to unexpected situations (think recovering from a near-stumble). And remember, change doesn't need to be massive! Even small modifications to your favorite stability exercises can make a significant impact over time.

Modify for Success

As you build stability and strength, it's crucial to keep your workouts evolving to avoid plateaus. One effective strategy is to embrace the power of subtle changes. You don't always need a complete revamp – sometimes, minor tweaks can have a significant impact! Try slowing down your exercises to really feel that deep muscle burn, or narrow your stance to add a balance challenge. Want to push further? Try those same familiar exercises with your eyes closed (do this safely!), forcing your core and stabilizing muscles to work extra hard.

Another fantastic resource as you progress is a physical therapist. They're your personalized coaches! A therapist can analyze your movements, identify any areas that need extra focus, and recommend exercise variations designed specifically for your current abilities.

But most importantly, listen to your body! It's your best guide on this journey. If an exercise feels too easy, it probably is. Find a way to make it more challenging. On the flip side, if a new variation causes knee pain, that's a red flag. Stop and either go back to an easier version or talk to a professional before continuing.

Remember, progress and protecting your knees go hand-in-hand. By staying adaptable, making small adjustments, and listening carefully to your body's signals, you'll continue to build strength and stability with confidence.

The Role of Professional Guidance

Expert Guidance: Key to Safe & Effective Exercise

There are many exercise tips and videos on the Internet, but again, you can't get all the nuances without that one-on-one attention that's critical for your knees. This is where a good physical therapist or knowledgeable trainer becomes indispensable. Besides being exercise gurus, they have an intrinsic understanding of body mechanics and can identify issues at their roots.

At Innovative Nerve & Joint Centers, our team is particularly well-equipped to help you construct a superior stability program. We'll identify precisely where your imbalances and movement limitations lie, along with any weakness contributing to your knee issues. Your individualized program will include exercises to correct them, plus a plan to build all-over strength and support that will maintain healthy knees.

We can give you the knowledge, tools, and hands-on adjustments so you can exercise safely and effectively. We will do all we can to empower you to reach your health goals, ease discomfort, and regain confidence to get back to the things you love.

DIY vs. Pro: Which Exercise Approach Is Right?

Forget those endless internet searches for the "right" exercises! A personalized plan eliminates the guesswork. Your physical therapist or trainer will carefully choose exercises specifically designed to target your weaknesses and help you achieve your individual goals. This focused approach saves you time and ensures you're making the most of your workouts.

Proper form isn't just about gym aesthetics – it's about getting results and protecting yourself from injury. An expert eye can spot those subtle mistakes in your technique that might be sabotaging your progress or even putting strain on your knees. Their guidance gives you confidence that you're moving in ways that truly benefit your body.

Sometimes, the smallest adjustments can make the biggest difference. A professional might suggest a slightly narrower stance to bring more balance work into your squat, or ask you to slow down your exercise tempo to really feel those deep core muscles engage. This kind of fine-tuning is what can take your results to the next level and often leads to faster progress than figuring it out on your own.

Let's be honest, even the most dedicated person has days where motivation takes a nosedive. Having regular check-ins with a therapist or trainer provides a powerful dose of accountability. They'll help you stay consistent, push through those challenging times, and celebrate your wins along the way!

Finding Your Team: Building Strength with a Professional

Choosing the right professional to guide your stability journey is just as important as the exercises themselves. Here's how to find someone who'll be a true partner in your knee health:

- **Seek Out Specialists:** Look for physical therapists or trainers who have specific expertise in knee health or rehabilitation. Our team at Innovative Nerve & Joint Centers specializes in treating knee pain. We understand the intricacies of the knee joint and design programs that address not only your current issues but also help prevent future problems.
- **Tap into Your Network:** Ask your doctor or friends who've had successful rehab journeys, or even search reputable online resources for recommendations. Word-of-mouth can be a great way to find professionals with a positive track record.

- **The Interview:** That initial consultation is crucial! Don't hesitate to ask about their experience with clients similar to you, their overall approach to knee stability, and how they personalize their programs. The right fit is someone who makes you feel heard, understood, and motivated.

Remember, it's an investment in YOU! Working with a knowledgeable professional like those at Innovative Nerve & Joint Centers is an investment in your knee health, both for the immediate challenges you're facing and for your long-term well-being. We'll provide personalized advice, targeted exercises, and ongoing support to manage and heal your knee pain quickly, empowering you to get back to the activities you enjoy.

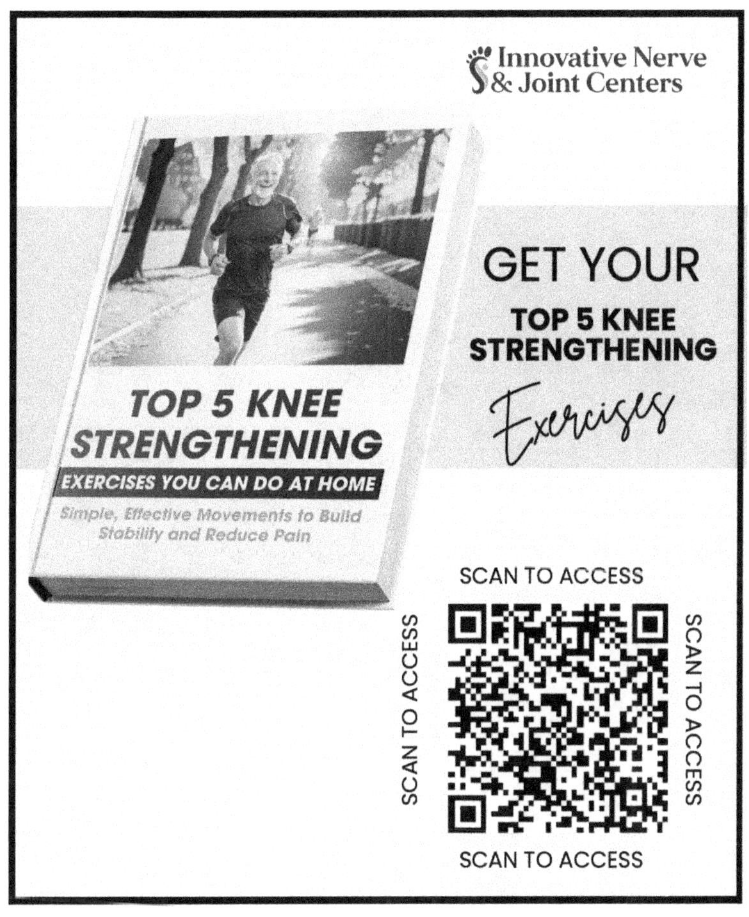

Unlock Your Path To Knee Pain Relief Now: Call (833) 359-6099 To Speak With An Expert Today!

8

KNEE PAIN AND MENTAL HEALTH

Lisa, a retired teacher, sat in my office, tears welling up in her eyes. It wasn't just the physical pain in her knee that brought her to tears; it was the emotional weight of it all. "I used to be so active," she explained, her voice trembling, "I loved hiking, gardening, spending time with my grandchildren. Now, I can barely walk to the mailbox without feeling excruciating pain." Lisa's knee pain had not only limited her physical abilities but had also stolen her joy, leaving her feeling isolated and depressed. She'd lost interest in her hobbies and avoided social gatherings, afraid of being a burden.

Lisa's story wasn't just about a physical ailment; it was a testament to the profound emotional toll chronic pain can take. The FREEDOM Protocol, I explained, addresses not just the physical aspects of knee pain but also the emotional and mental health challenges that often accompany it. As we worked together, Lisa's personalized plan incorporated not only targeted exercises and therapies but also stress management techniques like mindfulness and meditation. We encouraged her to connect with our support group, finding solace and strength in shared experiences. As Lisa progressed, I reminded her that everyone's healing journey is unique, and her experience isn't necessarily representative of what others might achieve.

Months later, a transformed Lisa walked into my office, a genuine smile radiating from her face. "I feel like myself again," she shared, "I'm gardening, spending time with my family, and I even joined a hiking group! The pain isn't completely gone, but I have the tools to manage it, and that's made all the difference." Now, not everyone will experience these same benefits, but Lisa's story is a powerful reminder of the intricate connection between our physical and emotional well-being.

The Emotional Toll of Chronic Knee Pain

Knee pain isn't just a physical ailment; it casts a long shadow over your emotional well-being too. Chronic pain, like the kind that often accompanies knee issues, can seep into every corner of your life, affecting your mood, relationships, and overall quality of life. It's important to acknowledge that the emotional impact of knee pain is just as real and significant as the physical discomfort.

The Link Between Knee Pain and Mental Health Conditions

Research has shown a strong correlation between chronic pain and mental health conditions like depression and anxiety. The constant discomfort, sleep disturbances, and limitations on daily activities can take a toll on your emotional resilience. Pain can drain your energy, making it difficult to engage in activities you once enjoyed, leading to feelings of sadness, frustration, and even isolation.

This often creates a vicious cycle: pain worsens mental health, and emotional distress amplifies pain perception. When you're feeling down or anxious, your body's natural pain-coping mechanisms may become less effective, making the pain feel even more intense. Breaking this cycle is crucial for managing both your knee pain and your emotional well-being.

Common Emotional Challenges Associated with Knee Pain

Knee pain can trigger a wide range of emotions, and it's important to recognize and validate these feelings. Some common emotional challenges include:

- **Frustration and Anger:** It's natural to feel frustrated when pain limits your ability to do the things you love. You might feel angry at your body for betraying you or resentful of others who don't understand your struggles.
- **Sadness and Grief:** Chronic pain can lead to a sense of loss – the loss of physical abilities, independence, and the life you once knew. It's okay to grieve these losses and allow yourself to feel the sadness.
- **Anxiety and Worry:** The uncertainty of chronic pain can fuel anxiety and worry. You might constantly worry about the future, fearing that the pain will worsen or that you'll become more disabled.
- **Social Isolation and Withdrawal:** Pain can make it difficult to socialize and participate in activities you once enjoyed. This can lead to feelings of isolation and loneliness, further impacting your emotional well-being.

Understanding these emotional challenges is the first step towards addressing them. Remember, you're not alone in this journey. Many people with knee pain experience similar emotional struggles. Seeking support from loved ones, healthcare professionals, or support groups can make a significant difference in your emotional well-being and your ability to cope with chronic pain.

Coping Strategies for Emotional Well-being

When knee pain becomes a daily struggle, it's easy to feel overwhelmed and discouraged. The emotional toll of chronic pain can be just as debilitating as the physical discomfort. But remember, you're not alone, and there are effective strategies to help you cope with the emotional challenges and regain control of your well-being.

Seeking Professional Help

Don't hesitate to reach out for professional support if you're struggling to manage the emotional impact of knee pain. Mental health professionals specializing in chronic pain can provide invaluable guidance and tools to navigate this challenging journey.

- **The Importance of Mental Health Support:** Therapists, counselors, and psychologists can help you understand and process the complex emotions associated with chronic pain. They can teach you coping mechanisms, stress-reduction techniques, and strategies for improving your overall well-being.

- **Cognitive-Behavioral Therapy (CBT):** This evidence-based therapy focuses on identifying and challenging negative thought patterns that can exacerbate pain and emotional distress. CBT equips you with practical skills to manage pain, reduce anxiety, and improve your mood.
- **Support Groups:** Connecting with others who are going through similar experiences can be incredibly empowering. Support groups provide a safe space to share your struggles, gain insights from others, and receive encouragement and understanding.

Self-Care Practices

Taking care of your emotional well-being is just as important as caring for your physical health. Incorporating self-care practices into your daily routine can help you manage stress, improve your mood, and build resilience.

- **Mindfulness and Meditation:** These practices involve focusing your attention on the present moment and accepting your thoughts and feelings without judgment. Mindfulness and meditation can help reduce stress, anxiety, and pain perception. Even a few minutes of daily practice can make a significant difference.

- **Journaling:** Writing down your thoughts and feelings can be a therapeutic way to process emotions and gain insights into your pain triggers and coping mechanisms. It can also help you track your progress and identify patterns in your pain experience.

- **Creative Outlets:** Engaging in creative activities like painting, drawing, writing, or playing music can provide a healthy outlet for emotional expression and stress relief. These activities can also help you connect with your inner self and find joy and meaning in life, even amidst the challenges of chronic pain.

- **Physical Activity:** While it might seem counterintuitive, gentle exercise can be beneficial for both your physical and emotional health. Even low-impact activities like walking, swimming, or tai chi can release endorphins, improve mood, and reduce stress. Be sure to consult with your doctor or physical therapist to determine safe and appropriate exercises for your specific condition.

Building a Support Network

You don't have to face the challenges of knee pain alone. Building a strong support network can provide you with the encouragement, understanding, and practical help you need to navigate this journey.

- **Talking to Loved Ones:** Share your experiences and feelings with your family and friends. Let them know how they can support you, whether it's through a listening ear, practical help with daily tasks, or simply spending time together.
- **Joining Online Communities:** Connect with others who are living with knee pain through online forums or social media groups. These communities can offer valuable information, support, and a sense of belonging.
- **Seeking Support from Healthcare Providers:** Your doctors, therapists, and other healthcare providers are valuable resources for emotional support. Don't hesitate to discuss your emotional challenges with them. They can offer guidance, connect you with mental health professionals, or adjust your treatment plan to better address your needs.

Taking care of your emotional well-being is an essential part of managing chronic knee pain. By seeking professional help, practicing self-care, and building a strong support network, you can navigate the emotional challenges of knee pain and improve your overall quality of life.

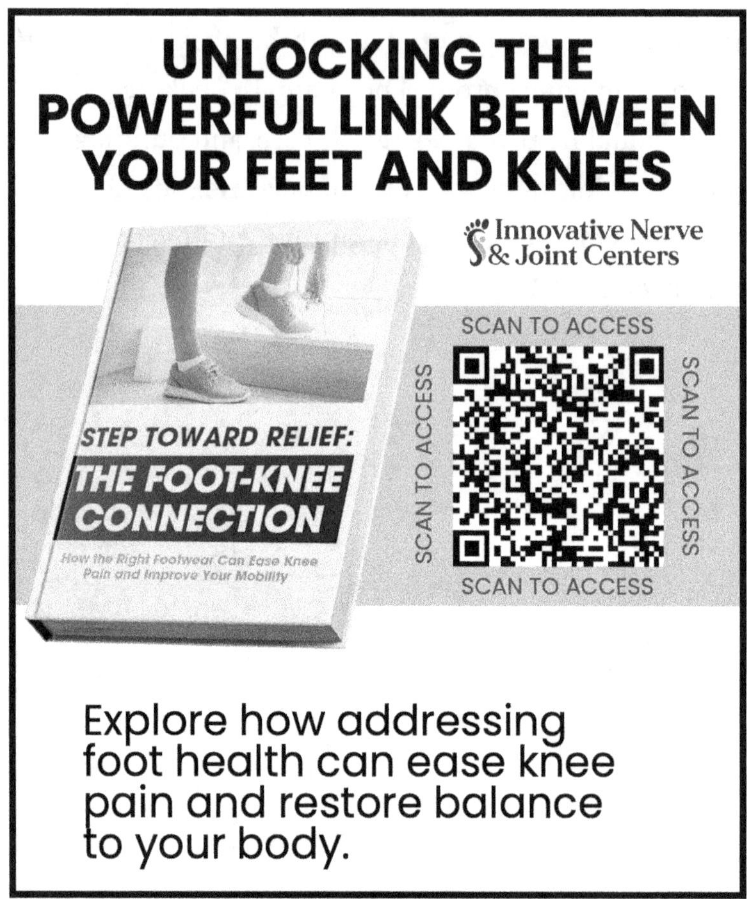

Unlock Your Path To Knee Pain Relief Now: Call (833) 359-6099 To Speak With An Expert Today!

9

THE IMPORTANCE OF PROPER FOOTWEAR AND ORTHOTICS

Sally, a vibrant yoga instructor, hobbled into my office, her usual energetic bounce replaced by a grimace. "My knee pain is getting worse," she explained, wincing as she sat down. "It's affecting my ability to teach, and I'm worried I'll have to give up the practice I love." Sally depended on her body for her livelihood, and her knee pain was threatening not only her career but also her passion. She'd tried various shoe inserts and even considered giving up yoga altogether, a thought that brought a shadow of sadness to her eyes.

During Sally's assessment, I noticed something interesting about her footwear. She was wearing trendy, minimalist shoes that offered little support or cushioning. Her arches were collapsing inward with each step, putting undue stress on her knees. We discussed the importance of proper footwear, explaining how seemingly insignificant choices can significantly impact knee health. As part of her FREEDOM Protocol plan, we recommended supportive shoes with custom orthotics designed to address her specific foot mechanics and gait pattern. We also incorporated exercises to strengthen her feet and ankles, improving stability and alignment. I cautioned Sally that the results of incorporating custom orthotics can vary greatly from person to person.

Months later, Sally practically danced into my office, her energy restored. "I can't believe the difference the orthotics have made!" she exclaimed. "My knee pain is practically gone, and I'm back to teaching full-time. I feel grounded and supported, both on and off the mat." *Your results may be different.* Sally's transformation highlighted the often-overlooked connection between our feet and our knees.

Your Feet: The Foundation of Knee Health

Your feet are the unsung heroes of your body, tirelessly supporting your weight and propelling you through life's adventures. But did you know that they also play a crucial role in the health of your knees? It's true! Your feet and knees are intimately connected, forming a kinetic chain that influences your entire body's alignment and movement.

Think of your feet as the foundation of a building. If the foundation is uneven or unstable, the entire structure is compromised. Similarly, if your feet aren't functioning optimally, it can throw off the alignment of your knees, leading to pain, discomfort, and even injury.

Common Foot Problems That Contribute to Knee Pain

Several common foot problems can wreak havoc on your knees. Let's take a closer look at some of the main culprits:

- **Overpronation (Flat Feet):** If you have flat feet, your arches collapse excessively when you walk or run. This causes your feet to roll inward (pronate) more than they should, which can twist your lower leg and put stress on the inner side of your knee. Over time, this can lead to pain and inflammation in the medial (inner) knee structures.
- **Supination (High Arches):** On the other end of the spectrum, high arches can also cause problems. If your arches are too high, your feet don't roll inward enough, leading to instability

and excessive pressure on the outer side of your foot and knee. This can irritate the lateral (outer) knee structures and contribute to pain and dysfunction.

- **Other Foot Conditions:** Bunions (bony bumps at the base of your big toe), hammertoes (bent toes), and plantar fasciitis (inflammation of the tissue that runs along the bottom of your foot) can all alter your gait and foot mechanics, indirectly affecting your knee alignment and function.

Understanding how your feet impact your knees is crucial for preventing and managing knee pain. By addressing any underlying foot problems, you can improve your overall alignment, reduce stress on your knees, and pave the way for a more active, pain-free life.

Supportive Footwear: Your First Line of Defense

Your shoes are more than just a fashion statement; they're the unsung heroes of your knee health. The right footwear can make a world of difference in preventing knee pain, managing existing discomfort, and improving your overall mobility. Let's explore the crucial role shoes play in safeguarding your knees:

- **Providing Cushioning and Shock Absorption:** Every step you take sends shockwaves through your body, and your knees bear the brunt of this impact. Supportive shoes with adequate cushioning act as shock absorbers, dissipating these forces and reducing the stress on your knee joints. This is especially important for activities like running or jumping, where the impact is even greater.

- **Offering Stability and Support:** Your feet and ankles play a crucial role in maintaining proper knee alignment. Supportive shoes with features like sturdy heels and arch support help keep your feet in a neutral position, preventing excessive rolling inward (overpronation) or outward (supination). This, in turn, promotes better knee alignment, reducing the risk of pain and injury.

- **Correcting Gait Abnormalities:** If you have a tendency to overpronate or supinate, specialized shoes can help correct these gait abnormalities. Motion control shoes are designed to limit excessive inward rolling, while stability shoes provide a balance of support and flexibility for those with mild to moderate overpronation. For individuals with high arches, cushioned shoes with ample flexibility can help promote a more natural gait pattern.

Choosing the Right Shoes for Your Needs

Selecting the right footwear is a crucial step in maintaining knee health and preventing pain. It's not just about finding a stylish pair; it's about choosing shoes that provide the support, cushioning, and stability your feet and knees need to thrive.

- **Activity-Specific Footwear:** Different activities place different demands on your feet and knees. Wearing shoes designed for your specific activity can significantly reduce the risk of injury and discomfort.
  - **Walking Shoes:** Look for shoes with flexible soles, ample cushioning, and a comfortable fit. They should provide good arch support and a roomy toe box to allow your toes to spread naturally.
  - **Running Shoes:** Running shoes need to offer more cushioning and shock absorption than walking shoes to handle the repetitive impact of running. They should also provide stability to control

excessive foot motion and reduce stress on your knees.

- Cross-Training Shoes: If you participate in a variety of activities, cross-training shoes offer a versatile option. They provide a balance of support, cushioning, and flexibility to accommodate different movements.

- Other Activities: If you engage in sports like basketball, tennis, or hiking, choose shoes specifically designed for those activities. These shoes will offer the features and support needed to handle the unique demands of each sport.

- **Foot Type Considerations:** Your foot type plays a significant role in determining the right shoes for you.

   - Low Arches (Flat Feet): If you have flat feet, you'll need shoes with motion control features to limit excessive inward rolling (overpronation). Look for shoes with sturdy heels, firm midsoles, and straight lasts (the shape of the shoe).

   - Neutral Arches: If you have neutral arches, you have a balanced stride and don't need as much motion control. Stability shoes

with moderate support and cushioning are
a good option.

- ○ **High Arches:** If you have high arches, your
  feet don't roll inward enough, which can
  lead to instability. Choose cushioned shoes
  with ample flexibility to encourage a more
  natural gait pattern.

- **Fit and Comfort:** No matter your activity or
  foot type, proper fit is essential. Shoes that are
  too tight or too loose can cause blisters,
  pressure points, and other foot problems that
  can affect your knee function. When trying on
  shoes, make sure there's enough room in the
  toe box for your toes to wiggle, and ensure that
  your heel doesn't slip out of the back of the
  shoe. Walk around in the shoes to assess their
  comfort and support before making a
  purchase.

By considering these factors and investing in the right
footwear, you're taking a proactive step towards
protecting your knees and ensuring a lifetime of pain-
free movement. Remember, your feet are the
foundation of your body, and taking care of them is
essential for overall health and well-being.

Custom Orthotics: Personalized Support for Your Feet

Think of custom orthotics as the tailored suit of the footwear world. While off-the-shelf shoe inserts offer general support, custom orthotics are crafted specifically for your unique feet and gait patterns. They're like a personal trainer for your feet, guiding them into proper alignment and optimizing their function.

What are Orthotics?

Orthotics are shoe inserts that are custom-made to fit your feet precisely. They're typically crafted from materials like plastic, foam, or graphite, and they can be designed to address a wide range of foot and ankle issues. Unlike generic insoles, custom orthotics are created based on a detailed assessment of your foot structure, gait mechanics, and individual needs.

The Benefits of Custom Orthotics for Knee Pain

Custom orthotics can be a game-changer for individuals struggling with knee pain, especially when the pain stems from biomechanical issues in the feet. Here's how they work their magic:

- **Improved Alignment:** By gently correcting misalignments in your feet and ankles, custom orthotics can promote better knee alignment. This reduces abnormal stress on the knee joint, which can alleviate pain and prevent further damage.

- **Reduced Stress on Joints:** Orthotics redistribute pressure more evenly across your feet, minimizing strain on specific areas that may be contributing to knee pain. This can be particularly beneficial for individuals with conditions like flat feet or high arches, where certain areas of the foot bear excessive weight.

- **Enhanced Shock Absorption:** Custom orthotics often incorporate materials that provide additional cushioning and shock absorption. This can be especially helpful for athletes and active individuals who engage in high-impact activities, as it reduces the force transmitted to the knees with each step.

- **Increased Comfort and Support:** By providing personalized support and addressing underlying foot problems, custom orthotics can significantly improve overall foot function and comfort. This can lead to reduced pain, improved mobility, and a better quality of life.

When to Consider Custom Orthotics

Custom orthotics are not a one-size-fits-all solution, but they can be a valuable tool for many individuals experiencing knee pain. Here are some scenarios where custom orthotics might be worth considering:

- **Chronic Knee Pain:** If you've tried conservative treatments like physical therapy, medication, or shoe modifications without sufficient relief, custom orthotics might offer a new avenue for pain management.
- **Specific Foot Conditions:** If you have flat feet, high arches, bunions, hammertoes, or other biomechanical issues, custom orthotics can help correct these problems and alleviate the resulting knee pain.
- **Athletes and Active Individuals:** If you engage in activities that put significant stress on your knees, such as running, jumping, or court sports, custom orthotics can provide additional support and protection, reducing your risk of injury.

If you're considering custom orthotics, it's important to consult with a qualified healthcare professional, such as a podiatrist or physical therapist. They can assess your individual needs, conduct a thorough evaluation of your feet and gait, and recommend the most appropriate type of orthotic for your specific situation.

Working with a Foot and Ankle Specialist

While the idea of custom orthotics might sound appealing, it's crucial to consult with a foot and ankle specialist before diving in. These experts, such as podiatrists, have the knowledge and tools to assess your individual needs and determine if orthotics are the right solution for you.

The Importance of Professional Assessment

A professional assessment is the cornerstone of getting custom orthotics that truly work. This evaluation goes beyond simply looking at your feet; it's a comprehensive analysis of your foot structure, gait mechanics, and any underlying issues that might be contributing to your knee pain.

During the assessment, the specialist will typically:

- **Examine Your Feet:** They'll check for any abnormalities in your foot structure, such as flat feet, high arches, bunions, or hammertoes.
- **Analyze Your Gait:** They'll observe how you walk or run, looking for any imbalances,

asymmetries, or unusual movement patterns that could be putting stress on your knees.

- **Discuss Your Symptoms and Medical History:** They'll ask about your knee pain, any previous injuries, and any other relevant medical conditions.

Based on this comprehensive assessment, the specialist can determine if custom orthotics are likely to benefit you and, if so, what type of orthotic would be most appropriate for your specific needs.

The Process of Getting Custom Orthotics

If custom orthotics are recommended, the process typically involves the following steps:

1. **Comprehensive Foot and Gait Analysis:** This in-depth evaluation involves examining your feet, observing your gait, and possibly using specialized tools like pressure plates or video analysis to assess your foot mechanics in detail.

2. **Casting or Scanning of Your Feet:** To create a precise mold of your feet, the specialist will either take a physical cast of your feet using plaster or foam, or use a 3D scanner to create a digital model.

3. **Custom Fabrication of Orthotics:** Using the cast or scan, a skilled technician will create your custom orthotics. The materials and design will be tailored to your specific needs, addressing any biomechanical issues identified during the assessment.

Follow-Up Care and Adjustments

Once you receive your custom orthotics, it's important to follow up with your specialist to ensure they fit properly and are functioning as intended. You may need to wear them gradually to allow your feet to adjust, and minor adjustments may be necessary to optimize their effectiveness.

It's important to note that custom orthotics are not a quick fix. They are a therapeutic tool that can provide significant benefits for knee pain when used in conjunction with other treatments like physical therapy and exercise. By working with a qualified foot and ankle specialist and following their recommendations, you can maximize the effectiveness of your orthotics and take a proactive step towards a pain-free, active life.

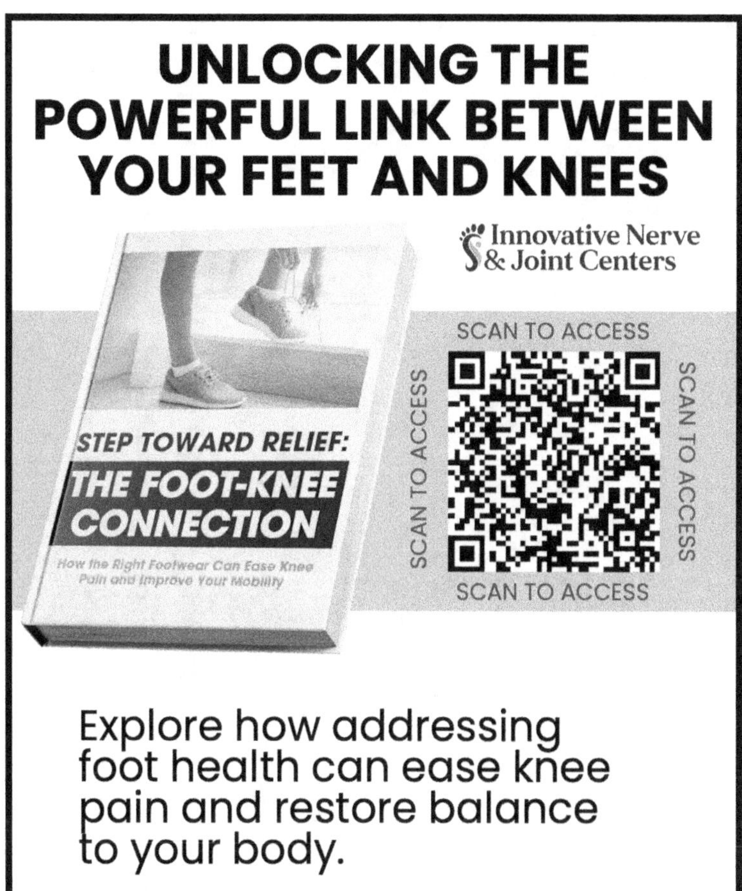

Unlock Your Path To Knee Pain Relief Now: Call (833) 359-6099 To Speak With An Expert Today!

10

VARIABLE TREATMENT PLANS FOR OPTIMIZED RESULTS

John, a retired firefighter, walked into my office with a determined glint in his eyes. "I want to hike the Appalachian Trail," he declared, "but this knee pain is holding me back." John's dream, though ambitious, was deeply personal. He saw it as a way to challenge himself physically and mentally, a testament to his resilience after a demanding career. He'd tried various treatments, but his knee pain persisted, making even short walks uncomfortable. He was beginning to lose hope that his dream would ever become a reality.

John's initial assessment revealed a complex picture: osteoarthritis in one knee, a previous meniscus tear in the other, and significant muscle imbalances throughout his lower body. A one-size-fits-all approach wouldn't cut it. With the FREEDOM Protocol, we crafted a dynamic treatment plan, adapting and adjusting as we went along. We started with gentle exercises to improve his range of motion and reduce inflammation. As his strength and mobility increased, we incorporated more challenging exercises, mimicking the demands of hiking. We also addressed his nutritional needs and incorporated stress management techniques to support his overall well-being. I explained to John that his progress might not always be linear, and setbacks, while frustrating, are opportunities to learn and refine the treatment plan. His success, however inspiring, is not a guarantee for others. Individual results may vary.

Months later, John sent me a picture from the Appalachian Trail, beaming, his trekking poles planted firmly on the ground. He was living his dream, one step at a time. His journey illustrates the core principle of the FREEDOM Protocol:

Adapting to Each Patient's Journey

The FREEDOM Difference: Tailored Treatment, Every Step of the Way

At the heart of the FREEDOM Protocol lies a fundamental understanding: no two patients are alike, and neither should their treatment plans be. Your knee pain, your goals, your body's unique way of healing – all of these factors shape your journey toward optimal health. That's why rigid, one-size-fits-all approaches often fall short. The FREEDOM program sets itself apart with treatment plans that are intentionally flexible, and designed to evolve alongside your progress.

The Art of Personalized Care

Imagine your treatment plan as a custom-tailored roadmap, complete with the option for scenic detours along the way. This isn't about following a predetermined set of directions. It's about honoring the fact that you are an individual, with a story that has shaped your current knee health.

Think about the factors that make up your unique picture:

- **Your Injury History**: Was your knee pain triggered by a specific incident, or has it crept up gradually? Old injuries, even seemingly minor ones, can leave lingering weaknesses that contribute to current problems.
- **Movement Patterns**: How you move matters. Subtle imbalances in the way you walk, run, or

squat can put excess strain on your knees. Your treatment plan might incorporate exercises focused on changing these long-ingrained patterns.

- **Beyond the Knee:** Knee health isn't isolated. Your hip strength, ankle mobility, even your posture, can all play a role. A truly personalized plan looks at your body as a whole system.
- **Lifestyle:** Are you a weekend warrior pushing yourself too hard? Is your job physically demanding? Do you spend long hours sitting? Your lifestyle habits significantly impact your joints and how well your body recovers.

Understanding these pieces of your puzzle is what allows us to create a treatment plan that truly targets the root causes of your knee pain, not just the surface-level symptoms. A generic knee strengthening program won't address the unique combination of factors contributing to your pain. But with a personalized plan, we can create a strategy as unique as you are, giving you the greatest chance for lasting success.

Dynamic Bodies, Dynamic Plans

The beauty of the FREEDOM program is that it understands your body isn't static; neither should your treatment plan be. Progress is rarely a perfectly straight line. Let's explore some scenarios:

- You came in hesitant, fearful of pain limiting your life. But those initial exercises are working wonders – you're moving more easily, and pain is fading. This isn't the time to stick to the original slow-and-steady plan. We might accelerate things, introducing tougher variations, integrating balance challenges, helping you re-discover the joy of movement faster than you imagined.

- You've been consistent, but suddenly a flare-up throws a wrench in the works. This doesn't mean failure. It's a signal that your plan needs a temporary detour. We might dial back the intensity, switch to gentler pain-relief techniques, and focus on maintaining the strength you've already built while we pinpoint what triggered the setback.

- The Unexpected Breakthrough: Sometimes, a small exercise adjustment makes a world of difference. Maybe a minor tweak in your form unlocks a new level of stability, or suddenly you're able to squat deeper without pain. We seize those opportunities! This might mean adding more demanding exercises or revising your timeline to reach your goals sooner.

This constant evolution of your plan is what sets the FREEDOM program apart. We don't just treat your knee in isolation; we treat you, the whole person. Your plan adapts because you do, optimizing your results and keeping setbacks from derailing your progress.

The Science of Adaptability

Flexibility isn't just about being accommodating; it's rooted in a deep understanding of how your body functions and heals. Understanding that healing takes time is crucial. It's not a straight, steady climb to recovery. Think of tissue healing happening in stages: first, there's inflammation, then repair, and finally a remodeling phase. Your treatment plan needs to adapt to those stages. Trying to push too hard in the early inflammation stage can worsen the problem, whereas introducing targeted exercises at the right point in the healing process speeds things up.

It's also important to acknowledge that knee pain isn't a simple equation – more damage doesn't always equal more pain. Inflammation, protective muscle tightness, and even how sensitive your nervous system is, all play a role in the pain you feel. This means your treatment plan might sometimes prioritize calming things down and reducing pain signals, rather than just focusing on building strength.

Your knee isn't an island! It's part of a complex system of movement, with your hips, ankles, and core all playing supporting roles. Understanding how your knee moves and the forces it withstands (that's biomechanics!) is essential. A treatment plan that includes exercises focused on movement quality isn't just about fixing what hurts now; it's about preventing future injury and truly optimizing your knee health.

Lastly, the FREEDOM method recognizes the mind-body connection. Your stress levels, sleep patterns, and emotional well-being all impact your pain and how quickly your body heals. That's why your plan might integrate relaxation techniques or other strategies to help you manage stress in addition to your physical exercises.

The Power of Variable Plans

Real Patients, Real Results: Midday Reflections

My midday consultations are a constant reminder of why the FREEDOM Protocol is so effective. It's where textbook knowledge translates into real-world results.

Each patient interaction reinforces the power of a treatment plan that's as flexible and multifaceted as the people it serves.

Beyond the Textbook Knee

While knee pain brings patients through the door, that's rarely the whole story. As we discuss their experiences, underlying factors emerge. Perhaps their hectic work life fuels stress, impacting their healing, or disrupted sleep patterns exacerbate their pain sensitivity. The FREEDOM approach isn't compartmentalized. It allows me to address these broader issues alongside the physical treatment – we might talk about quick stress-reducing techniques, or tips for creating a sleep-friendly environment. Healing occurs on many levels.

An Ounce of Prevention

Getting someone out of pain today is only half the victory. True success lies in equipping them with the tools to avoid future setbacks. As a patient progresses, we shift focus toward long-term resilience. This means incorporating exercises that address weaknesses common to knee injuries, teaching them how to move correctly to avoid unnecessary strain, and even discussing strategies to manage a flare-up if it happens down the road. This proactive approach empowers them to take ownership of their knee health.

The beauty of the FREEDOM program is that it understands people are complex. Pain, healing, and long-term well-being are influenced by a multitude of factors. A treatment plan that allows for those individual needs, adapting to both physical and lifestyle elements, is what leads to lasting, transformative change.

Navigating the Ups and Downs of Recovery

The journey toward knee health isn't always a smooth, predictable path. There will be great days that boost your motivation and some days where it feels like you're taking a few steps backward. This is where the adaptability of the FREEDOM method truly becomes your greatest asset.

Setbacks as Intel

Let's say a flare-up throws a wrench in your progress. Instead of getting discouraged, we see this as valuable information. Together, we try to figure out the trigger – did you overdo it one day? Is there a movement pattern that's causing irritation? Understanding the cause allows us to temporarily modify your plan. Maybe we dial down the intensity for a short period, or incorporate different exercises to calm an irritated knee. Setbacks become a tool for refining your path, not a roadblock.

Celebrating Victories, Big and Small

On the flip side, some patients experience incredibly rapid progress. This is a time to seize the momentum! Instead of blindly sticking to the original plan, we might ramp up the challenge, introduce new variations, and push those boundaries a little further. This keeps things both exciting and maximizes your potential at every stage.

The FREEDOM method embraces the reality that healing has a rhythm of its own. By having a treatment plan that can flex and flow with those changes, we can turn setbacks into learning opportunities, capitalize on those moments of rapid improvement, and ultimately keep you moving steadily toward your goals.

Your Path to Optimized Healing

Hope and Healing: Your Journey Starts Here

The stories I've shared – whether it's Sarah rediscovering the joy of hiking or John getting back to pain-free workouts – are not just examples. They're glimpses into a future that's possible for you, too. FREEDOM offers a path toward healing and hope because it's built on the understanding that your knee pain doesn't define you.

Embarking on Your Journey

If you're ready to take control of your knee health, to stop letting pain dictate your life, then the first step is simple: reach out to us at Innovative Nerve & Joint Centers. Our team is here to guide you through your personalized journey within the FREEDOM program. Here's what you can expect:

- **An initial consultation**: This is where we discuss your history, your goals, and create the foundation for your tailored plan.
- **Ongoing Adaptation**: As you progress, we will constantly assess, adjust, and celebrate those wins together.
- **Empowerment for the Long Run**: You'll leave equipped with the tools to maintain your knee health and prevent future setbacks.

You deserve to live a life unhindered by knee pain. We're ready to help you build a treatment plan as adaptable and resilient as you are. Call us at (833) 359-6099 or visit injcenters.com/contact to get started.

A Future of Mobility and Strength

Imagine a life where knee pain is a distant memory. Picture yourself confidently tackling those stairs, enjoying long walks, or even rediscovering a sport you thought you had to abandon. The FREEDOM Program isn't just about easing your current pain; it's about unlocking a future where your knees are a source of strength, not limitation. It's about reclaiming the active lifestyle you deserve.

Let's make that future a reality, together.

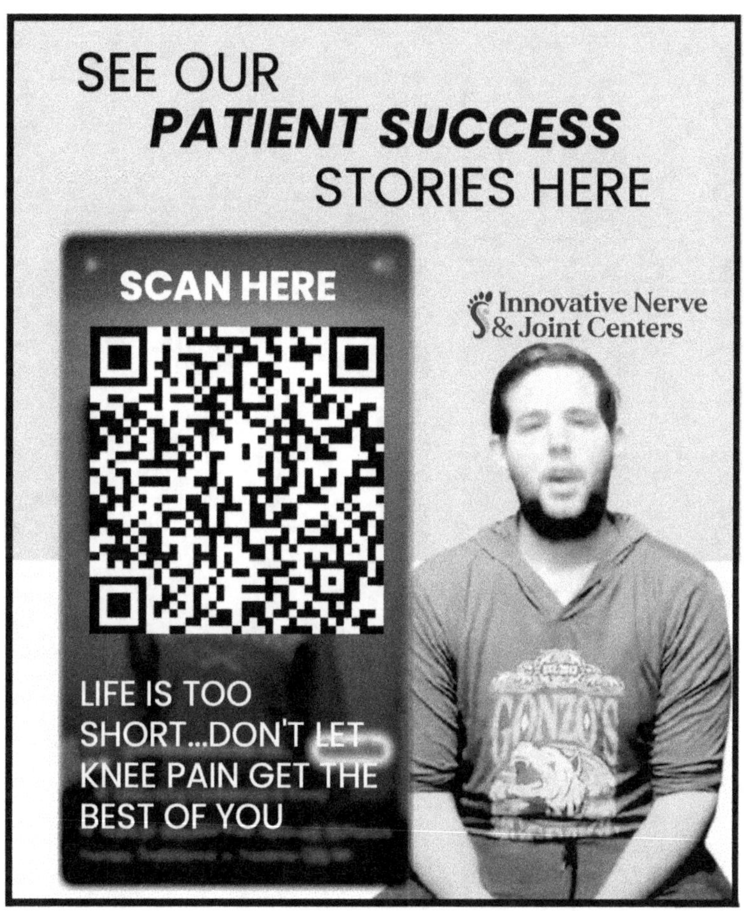

Unlock Your Path To Knee Pain Relief Now: Call (833) 359-6099 To Speak With An Expert Today!

11

YOUR PATH TO HEALING BEGINS HERE

You've journeyed through the pages of this book, learning about the intricacies of your knees, the root causes of pain, and the innovative approaches that can transform your life. Now, it's time to take that knowledge and embark on your own path to healing.

This chapter is your roadmap to freedom from knee pain. It's a culmination of everything you've learned so far, distilled into actionable steps you can take to reclaim your mobility, strength, and joy of movement. Whether you're just starting your healing journey or seeking to optimize your current approach, this chapter will guide you towards a brighter, pain-free future.

We'll recap the key principles of the FREEDOM Protocol, providing a clear and concise overview of the steps involved. We'll delve into practical tips for implementing these principles in your daily life, from creating a personalized exercise plan to optimizing your nutrition and managing stress. And we'll offer guidance on how to navigate the road to recovery, addressing common challenges and setbacks along the way.

Remember, healing is not a linear process. It's a journey with ups and downs, twists and turns. But with the right tools, support, and mindset, you can achieve lasting relief and reclaim your life from the grip of knee pain.

Success Stories: Lives Transformed

The walls of my office hold countless stories of transformation and renewed hope. But nothing motivates me more than seeing patients walk out my door with not just less pain, but a genuine spark back in their eyes. Here are just a few of those stories:

Chronic Pain to a Plan for Recovery: Katelyn's Journey

"After years of struggling with chronic pain, I finally feel like I have a road to recovery. Dr. Fisher doesn't just treat symptoms, he creates a personalized plan. His combination of laser therapy, physical therapy, and chiropractic care has made a significant difference in such a short time. I highly recommend this practice for anyone seeking lasting relief!"

From Pain to Renewed Mobility: Myriam's Experience

"Dr. Fisher and his team are incredible! I came in with back, neck, and knee pain, and within days, I felt a huge difference. I move more easily and truly feel younger. If you're struggling with pain, don't hesitate - they're amazing!"

From Constant Headaches to Lasting Relief: Ros's Success Story

"Dr. Fisher changed my life! My chronic headaches are now rare, something I never thought possible. Plus, when I needed knee surgery, he connected me with a great surgeon and provided fantastic physical therapy for a smooth recovery. He treats the whole person, not just the symptoms."

These are not just cases; they're individuals who bravely chose to fight for an active life. They are reminders of the profound difference the FREEDOM Protocol can make.

Why Choose the FREEDOM Protocol? It's the Difference That Delivers Results

You've likely tried other approaches for your knee pain, maybe with temporary relief but no lasting solution. That's because your knee pain is uniquely yours. The FREEDOM Protocol understands this, which is why it stands out from the rest:

- **Beyond Band-Aid Fixes**: Knee pain isn't just about the knee itself. It might stem from an old ankle sprain that subtly changed your gait, or from chronic inflammation in your body. Simply masking pain with pills or generic exercises won't fix those underlying issues. We dig deeper, finding the true source of your pain, giving you a true chance for lasting relief.
- **The Best of Both Worlds:** The FREEDOM program isn't afraid to innovate. Alongside tried-and-true physical therapy, we'll also incorporate cutting-edge techniques designed to improve circulation to your knee, calm down irritated nerves, or restore proper joint mechanics. This customized blend gives you the best possible chance of success.
- **Healing Takes More Than Exercise:** How you sleep, how you manage stress, even what you

eat – all of these can impact your joints. Our program looks at the whole picture, offering guidance to reduce inflammation, optimize your overall wellness, and create an environment where your knees can truly heal.

- **It Works! (Just Ask Our Patients):** Don't take our word for it. The testimonials you've read prove that the FREEDOM program has helped countless people reclaim their mobility and rediscover the joy of being active. If they can overcome their knee pain, so can you!

The FREEDOM method isn't just another set of exercises. It's a commitment to understanding your individual needs and empowering you with the tools, knowledge, and support to achieve long-term freedom from knee pain.

The First Step to Recovery: Your Initial Consultation

Your journey toward healing starts with understanding. That's why we begin with a comprehensive consultation and assessment. This isn't a rushed appointment; it's about giving us time to truly get to know you and your unique challenges.

We'll start with your story. We want to know about past injuries, how your knee pain impacts your daily life, and what you truly wish to achieve – is it pain-free walks? Hiking with your grandkids again? We tailor your plan according to those goals.

Next comes a thorough examination. We'll look at how you move – are there imbalances straining your knees? We'll assess your joint function and muscle strength to pinpoint specific weaknesses contributing to your pain.

From all this information, we'll work together to build your personalized treatment plan. This isn't a one-size-fits-all solution. We design exercises and therapies to directly address the areas we've identified as causing your pain. This is a collaboration because you are the expert on your own body. You'll have an active voice in shaping your path to recovery.

A Community of Support

At Innovative Nerve & Joint Centers, we believe healing is about more than just physical treatment. That's why we strive to create a true community of support. You're not alone in this battle against knee pain. Our dedicated team of professionals is invested in your success, offering guidance and encouragement every step of the way.

But the support doesn't end with us. Oftentimes, patients find an unexpected source of strength and connection in their fellow participants within the FREEDOM Protocol. Facing similar struggles fosters a sense of camaraderie. You might share tips that worked, offer a listening ear to someone having a tough day, or simply find comfort in knowing you're not in this alone. Together, as a community, we'll celebrate your victories, both big and small, on your journey toward reclaiming an active life.

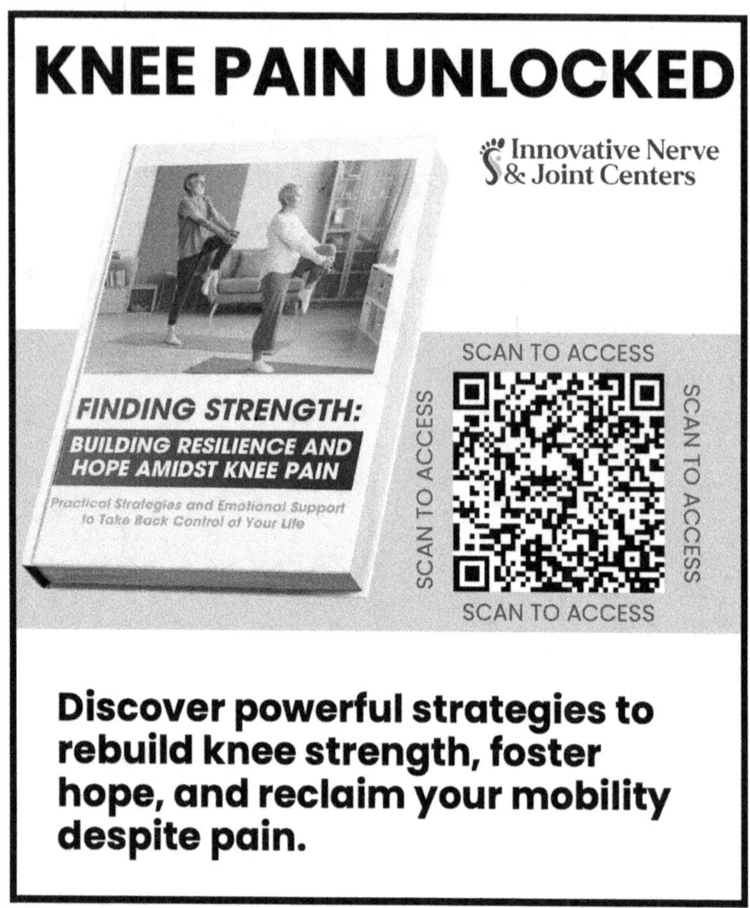

Unlock Your Path To Knee Pain Relief Now: Call (833) 359-6099 To Speak With An Expert Today!

12

CHOOSE ACTION, CHOOSE A LIFE OF FREEDOM

Emily, a vibrant grandmother, sat across from me, her eyes sparkling with a newfound joy. "I danced at my granddaughter's wedding!" she exclaimed, her voice filled with emotion. Just a few months prior, Emily had struggled to walk without pain, her knee osteoarthritis making even simple activities a challenge. She'd almost given up hope of ever dancing again, a pastime she'd cherished for years. She'd resigned herself to a life on the sidelines, watching her grandchildren play from a chair, her heart aching with the limitations her knee pain imposed.

Emily's journey with the FREEDOM Protocol was a testament to her resilience and the power of personalized care. Her customized plan addressed not only the physical aspects of her osteoarthritis but also the emotional toll it had taken. We combined targeted exercises, manual therapy, and nutritional guidance to reduce inflammation, improve joint function, and empower her to regain control of her life. While Emily experienced significant improvement, it's important to remember that individual results can vary. Emily's results are not guaranteed for everyone.

Emily's story, much like the countless others I've witnessed in my practice, underscores a powerful truth: a life free from knee pain is within reach. It's a choice, a decision to take action and embark on a journey of healing and transformation.

Congratulations on making it this far in the book! Your dedication to understanding and relieving your knee pain is truly inspiring. You've delved into the complexities of knee conditions, explored the limitations of conventional approaches, and discovered the potential for true, lasting healing through the FREEDOM Protocol. You now possess the knowledge, the seeds of transformation. But as the saying goes, knowledge without action is like a seed unplanted. It holds the promise of growth but remains dormant, its potential unrealized.

Are you ready to cultivate that potential? To nurture those seeds and watch them blossom into a life of greater mobility, strength, and joy?

If you're ready to take the next step, we invite you to schedule a consultation with us at Innovative Nerve & Joint Centers. This is your opportunity to embark on a personalized journey toward freedom from knee pain. During your consultation, we'll dive deeper into your unique situation, discuss your goals, and explore how the FREEDOM Protocol can help you achieve them. We'll answer your questions, provide personalized insights, and empower you to make informed decisions about your knee health. Please note that a consultation does not guarantee specific results. This is your chance to plant the seed, to take action, and to choose a life of FREEDOM.

For too long, knee pain may have felt like an inescapable sentence. Perhaps you've been told that surgery is inevitable, or that those twinges mean your active days are behind you. But I'm here to tell you that it doesn't have to be this way. Knee pain is not a life sentence. The FREEDOM Protocol exists because I believe in the body's potential to heal, and because countless patients have proven that transformation is possible. The choice is yours: accept the limitations, or take a bold step towards a different future.

Imagine this: stairs are no longer an obstacle, long walks are a pleasure, and you can finally bend down to play with your grandkids without wincing. The

FREEDOM Protocol isn't about a temporary fix, it's about unlocking the following:

- **Lasting Pain Reduction:** By addressing the root cause of your pain, we aim for significant and sustainable improvement, not just masking symptoms.
- **Reclaimed Mobility:** Strengthening the right muscles, restoring joint function – it translates into moving with greater ease and confidence.
- **Rediscovering Your Joy:** Whether it's hiking, gardening, or dancing, imagine getting back to the activities that bring you true joy.
- **The Support You Deserve:** This isn't a solo mission. You'll have expert guidance and a community cheering you on.

Now it's natural to have questions. Maybe you worry, "What if it doesn't work for me?" or "I don't have time for this." Let's address those concerns head-on:

- **Proven Results:** The testimonials you've read aren't anomalies. The FREEDOM method has a track record of success because it's based on sound principles and cutting-edge techniques.
- **Meeting You Where You Are:** Your treatment plan is tailored to your needs and lifestyle.

Worried about time commitment? We'll design a plan you can realistically follow.

- **No Failure, Just Feedback:** Healing isn't always linear. If we encounter setbacks, it's information, allowing us to adjust and refine your plan for better results.

Change starts with a single decision. If you're ready to say YES to a life less limited by knee pain, here's how to begin:

- **Call Innovative Nerve & Joint Centers:** Contact us at (833) 359-6099 to schedule your consultation or scan the code below to start your journey.

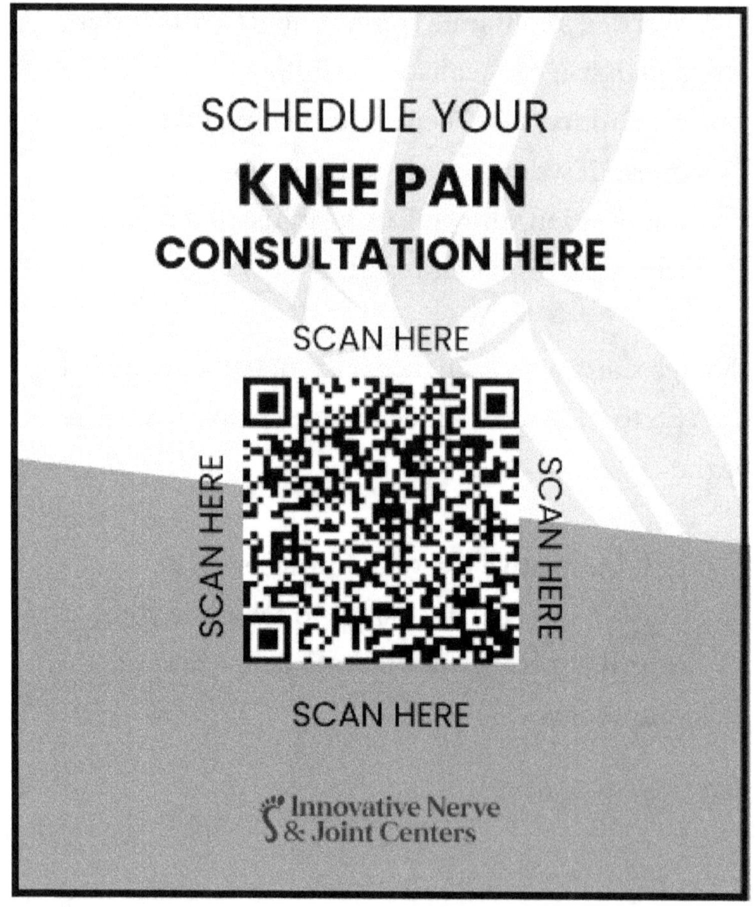

- **Free Masterclass:** Not near Chicago? Sign up for our free webinar, "Unveiling The Truth: 3 Breakthrough Secrets To Reversing Knee Pain," and learn more from the comfort of your home.

3 Secrets to
REVERSING
KNEE PAIN
MASTERCLASS
SCAN TO ACCESS
SCAN TO ACCESS
SCAN TO ACCESS
SCAN TO ACCESS
Innovative Nerve
& Joint Centers

Dance Again. Live Again. Start Today.

Our mission is simple: helping people like you overcome knee pain and reclaim a life of joy and movement. Just like Emily thought her dancing days were over because Knee pain kept her on the sidelines —watching life instead of living it. But after partnering with our clinic, she found herself twirling at her granddaughter's wedding, pain-free and full of joy. At our clinic, we don't just treat knees—we transform lives. With personalized plans, cutting-edge treatments, and a truly caring team, we're redefining what's possible for people like you. Ready to move better, feel better, and live better? Let's create your success story. Your next step? Simple:

Click below to book your one-on-one consultation. Let's get you back to doing what you love! Looking forward to meeting you and starting your healing journey.

Dr. Paul Fisher